The 21st Century is Making You Fat

The 21st Century is Making You Fat

Why your environment makes you put on weight and what you can do about it

Pat Thomas

GAIA
THINKING

An Hachette Livre UK Company

First published in Great Britain in 2008 by
Gaia, a division of Octopus Publishing Group Ltd
2–4 Heron Quays, London E14 4JP
www.octopusbooks.co.uk

ISBN 978-1-85675-290-9

A CIP catalogue record for this book is available from the British Library

Printed and bound in Italy

Printed on Cyclus Offset, a 100 per cent recycled paper

2 4 6 8 10 9 7 5 3 1

All reasonable care has been taken in the preparation of this book, but the
information it contains is not meant to take the place of medical care under the
direct supervision of a doctor. Before making any changes in your health regime,
always consult a suitably qualified doctor. Any application of the ideas and
information contained in this book is at the reader's sole discretion and risk.

Executive Editor: Sandra Rigby
Managing Editor: Clare Churly
Executive Art Editor: Darren Southern
Page make-up: Dorchester Typesetting Group Ltd
Senior Production Controller: Simone Nauerth

Contents

Acknowledgements   7

Introduction: A 21st-century problem   9

Chapter 1: How dieting fails us   15

Chapter 2: The bigger picture   37

Chapter 3: Sleep yourself thin   57

Chapter 4: The problem of 'chemical calories'   75

Chapter 5: Pills that make you plump   101

Chapter 6: The influence of allergies   121

Chapter 7: The stress factor   141

Chapter 8: You are what you eat   157

Chapter 9: A menu for permanent weight loss   185

Notes   210

Index   255

Acknowledgements

This book could not have been written without the support of family, friends and colleagues, all of whom have been prepared to tolerate my various absences – physical, mental and emotional. 'Wassup?!' to my son, Alex, and here's wishing that you inherit a healthier future. All praise to my agent Laura Longrigg, who, on my behalf, puts up with more than I probably ever know or acknowledge. Gratitude to Sandra Rigby and all at Gaia for recognizing the importance of this data in widening the ongoing debate about overweight and obesity. Special thanks to Paula Baillie-Hamilton, Professor Angelo Tremblay and Dr Leo Galland for their input. Love to my dear friends and colleagues at *The Ecologist* – the bravest people I know.

A 21st-century problem

This is not a diet book; I am not a diet guru. It is not about how to lose weight, so much as *why* we gain weight.

Even asking the question 'Why do we gain weight?' may seem ridiculous. Everyone knows that we gain weight because we eat too much. It's a simple equation, isn't it? If you eat more calories than you burn off, you get fat. So simple, in fact, that people who fail for one reason or another to lose weight must be either greedy or lazy.

Open a newspaper on any given day and you can usually find a story about the growing number of overweight and obese people throughout the UK and, indeed, the world. Obesity is now officially an 'epidemic'. Doctors are 'alarmed'; health officials are 'concerned'; and local authorities in every community, town and city are making a big noise about 'doing something' about it.

Obesity is a 21st-century problem – and the figures are shocking. Globally the prevalence of overweight and obesity has increased steadily since 1970.[1] The World Health Organization

9

has declared overweight as one of the top ten health risks in the world, and one of the top five in developed nations.[2] According to recent estimates, some 250 million people are clinically obese,[3] equivalent to 7 per cent of the adult population. Ironically, throughout the world the number of people who are overweight (estimated to be one billion) significantly outnumber those who are starving (estimated to be around 800 million).[4]

Obesity has serious long-term consequences for health. While it is not an immediately lethal disease, it plays a role in triggering or worsening a number of chronic – and sometimes serious – diseases and conditions,[5] including hypertension (high blood pressure), high cholesterol, heart disease, type-2 diabetes, gall-bladder disease, asthma, mental-health concerns (such as depression and low self-esteem) and joint and bone disorders.[6]

Being overweight or obese can also contribute to many problems in the female reproductive system, such as prolonged or heavy periods, menstrual pain, delayed ovulation, premenstrual syndrome, infertility, amenorrhoea (absence of menstruation), fibroids, tumours of the uterus, breast cancer, endometrial cancer, ovarian cancer and uterine prolapse.[7]

In the US, medical expenses for overweight and obesity accounted for 9.1 per cent of total US medical expenditure in 1998, costing around $78.5 billion.[8] In today's money that is more than $92 billion.

In the UK, 43 per cent of men and 34 per cent of women are overweight, and one in four adults and one in ten children under the age of 15 are obese.[9] The direct cost to the National Health Service (NHS) is £480 million. The indirect costs are estimated to be in the region of £2.5 billion per year, including costs to the NHS and those to industry caused through sickness and absence.

Most reports in the media trot out the same causes (the gluttony and sloth of modern society) and the same old solutions (eat less and exercise more).[10] And yet if weight loss were simply a matter of cutting calories and being more active, then the British population should be in pretty good shape. At any given time up to 50 per cent of the population in the UK is on a diet and/or an exercise regime. Worse, there is good data – as this book will show – that dietary regimes that severely restrict in the short term calories as well as food types (fats, carbohydrates and so on) actually encourage rebound weight gain over the longer term.[11]

Since there is not yet a medical cure for obesity, it is often easier to explain it away by blaming some weakness on the individual. Yet we know that simplistic solutions, such as eating less and/or exercising more, do not always produce results. Some theorists even believe that exercise contributes little to weight loss.[12] This is because physical activity accounts for a small proportion of an individual's total energy expenditure. About 80 per cent of one's energy is used to maintain the resting physiological processes of the body and to digest food.[13]

At the same time, individuals can vary enormously in the way they burn calories – something that conventional dieting wisdom finds hard to explain. And diet regimes have a shockingly high failure rate. In fact, depending upon how one reads the medical literature, conventional diet strategies have a success rate of just 3–7 per cent. Do the maths: this means that conventional weight-loss strategies have a failure rate of 93–97 per cent. Surely there is something more to obesity than simply eating too much or not exercising enough.

Clearly being overweight is a complex problem that cannot simply be explained away on a calories in/calories out basis. My own interest in the wider issues of this subject crept up on me. As an investigative journalist, I receive scientific studies (often in advance of publication) and see data that many mainstream

11

writers do not. For years I had been seeing reports trickling in of the connection between pollution and weight gain and associated illnesses such as diabetes and heart disease. I stored the data in a folder and kept a casual eye on developments.

Then, in 2005, newspapers in the UK printed a small story about a new 'fat map' of Britain. The map was drawn up and published by Dr Foster Intelligence, an independent health-research organization that works closely with the NHS and Experian, a market-research company.[14] The analysis was a synthesis of data from two different surveys – the Health Survey for England and the British Market Research Bureau's quarterly survey of 25,000 Britons – based on lifestyle and Body Mass Index details (BMI is a statistical indication of how overweight a person is; see pages 26–27) and geographical location. It found that people living in Britain's northern industrial towns were fatter than those living both in London and in other more rural areas.

Across the board the reportage was unremarkable. The results, after all, echoed those of previous studies and, having heard it all before, the newspapers avoided any original comment or analysis, focusing instead on the marvels of modern technology that enable us to pinpoint, down to a street, the places where the fattest people in the country live.

A quote from Dr Foster Intelligence about the threat of obesity, and the benefits of surveys like this one, made all the papers: 'We need to reduce levels of obesity, and detailed health maps like these show where the risks of obesity are highest,' commented the organization's marketing development manager, Dr Marc Farr. 'This will enable health authorities to target weight-loss drives in areas where this is a real problem ... Until now they have not had access to this accurate database, so this should make a difference.'[15]

Amazingly, data released at the same time in the US showed that there, too, people living in industrial towns also seemed to be carrying the most weight.[16]

The question that kept rattling around in my head was how does knowing *where* people are fattest make a dramatic difference to the problem of obesity? Surely the real question that needs answering is: *why* are we so fat? On this point, Farr hedged his bets and fell back on mainstream thinking, to conclude: 'The reasons for obesity [in these northern towns] are not uncommon and shared by many areas: availability of cheap, high-sugar food products, unemployment, age-related failure to engage in physical activity, understanding the nature and dangers of obesity and changes to more sedentary forms of employment.'

This oft-repeated explanation has some merit, of course, but it seemed to miss the vital point – which was shouting at me from my file of data – that the *where* and the *why* of being overweight are intricately linked.

So I wrote an article for *The Ecologist* magazine – and was universally pilloried for doing so. Conventional nutritionists, umbrella organizations that receive funding from the government to help fight obesity, and even a celebrity food writer came out of the woodwork. I was called naive and even a crackpot, not that any of them had bothered to read the evidence on the subject; it was just that what I had to say – that the pollution of a body with industrial chemicals can contribute to weight gain and make losing weight very difficult – was too new and contrary to everything they had been taught to believe.

The evidence, however, speaks for itself. Indeed, at the same time that my own article came out, a ground-breaking review by a panel of eminent scientists was also published, suggesting that evidence for the influence of what they called the 'Big Two' causes of obesity – overeating and underexercising – was circumstantial at best, and that other factors (see pages 38–55) needed to be taken into consideration if we were ever going to tackle effectively the problems of overweight and obesity.[17]

Many of these problems were, perhaps unsurprisingly, extensions of our 21st-century lifestyle, such as lack of sleep and exposure to industrial pollutants and even air conditioning. These recognized contributors to weight gain are what this book is all about, and if you have ever had trouble losing weight, you may find what it has to say both challenging and eye-opening. You may also find that the information contained here is empowering, and may even help you on the road towards a lifestyle that enables you to lose pounds gently, safely and permanently, in a way that leaves you healthier than you were before. If that is true for even one person, then this book will have been a success.

CHAPTER 1

How dieting fails us

You lose a few pounds; you gain back even more – it's a common experience for people who are fighting the battle of the bulge. Very low-calorie diets may bring quick results, but the weight loss can be difficult to maintain. And when the pounds pile on again, the finger of blame gets pointed squarely at the dieter: she 'cheated'; he got 'lazy'.

But while the propensity to 'cheat' or get 'lazy' occasionally lies within us all, the failure to lose weight and keep it off may not simply be a matter of failing to enforce an iron will. Increasingly scientific evidence shows that the low-calorie diet is, paradoxically, one of the main reasons why we find it so difficult to lose weight permanently.

In 2007, when researchers at the University of California, Los Angeles (UCLA), conducted a comprehensive and thorough analysis of 31 long-term studies of dieters, they found that although dieters can lose significant amounts of weight in the first few months, most will return to their starting weight within five years. Significantly the study, which was published in the journal *American Psychologist*, found that 83 per cent of people who go on diets eventually put on more weight than before they started.[1]

The researchers contentiously concluded that diets do not lead to sustained weight loss or health benefits for the majority of people, and that most of the people in these studies would have been better off not dieting at all, since their bodies would not suffer the tremendous wear and tear of losing weight and then gaining it all back. They rightly pointed to other evidence in numerous studies that a lifetime of repeatedly losing and then gaining weight has been linked to cardiovascular disease, strokes, diabetes and altered immune function.[2] Continual yo-yoing of weight also puts people at greater risk of dying prematurely.

Dieting and death aren't usually paired together. Indeed, most people are told that they need to diet in order to save their lives. But ignoring the evidence won't make the facts go away. For instance, the conclusions of an ongoing Nurses' Study[3] – one of the largest health studies ever conducted – are that women who have maintained a more or less stable weight since the age of 18 have the best prospects of a long life, free from health problems such as heart disease and strokes. This conclusion squares with several other research papers showing that fluctuating weight not only prevents long-term weight loss, but also damages the body's vital organs and can lead to a higher risk of early death.[4]

Read those first few paragraphs again: dieting doesn't work and isn't healthy. This may be the first time you have read such a statement; it may go against everything you have ever been led to believe. And yet the idea that dieting is the only way to lose weight is a perfect example of the principle that, if you say something often enough, it will become accepted as the truth – even if it isn't. Indeed, our obsession with dieting is perhaps best summed up by the old maxim that for every complex problem there is a simple answer – and it is usually wrong.

People who want to lose weight are now faced with a terrible contradiction. When society and the media tell us that thinner is better, and studies like the one at UCLA continue to show that diets don't work, it is time to take a look at the assumptions that underpin our thinking about dieting and health, and to broaden our far-too-narrow perspective on what makes us gain weight.

You can never be too thin ... or can you?

A large number of studies exist to show that gaining a moderate amount of weight in middle age may actually prolong life. Very underweight people may be more likely to die younger because they lack the reserves to withstand illness. Because of this, those who gain a moderate amount of weight (4.5–6.8 kg/10–15 lb) as they age may live longer.[5]

Some weight gain in middle age may even be protective. For post-menopausal women in particular, a little extra fat in middle age is the primary source of oestrogen production. This vital hormone not only protects the heart and bones, but also eases the characteristic symptoms of the menopause. Underweight women report significantly more menopausal symptoms than those who have allowed themselves to put on a moderate amount of weight.

It has long been known that lean women over the age of 50 have the greatest risk of suffering hip fractures – often as a result of osteoporosis (increased brittleness of the bones) – due to having less padding to absorb the shock of a fall. But experts now believe that weight loss after the menopause is also a significant risk factor.

In 1996 researchers at the National Institute on Aging in Maryland published the results of a study that followed 3,683 women who were at least 67 years old. The women were asked to recall their weight at the age of 50. Their weight changes and incidences of hip fractures were charted over eight years. All the women in the study who lost 10 per cent or more of their weight at the age of 50 doubled their chances of fracturing a hip. However, the increase was greatest for women who were already lean, who doubled their odds with a weight loss of just 5 per cent or more.[6]

In terms that most of us can understand, any gain under 10 kg (22 lb) through middle age is not significantly associated with an increased risk of early death. So the moral of the tale may be: moderation in all things – and moderation even in that. As a review of 13 reports from 11 diverse populations in the US and Europe concluded, '... the highest mortality rates occur in adults who either have lost weight or have gained excessive weight. The lowest mortality rates are generally associated with modest weight gain.'[7]

Calories in/calories out

Since the 1930s we have been held in thrall to the idea that weight loss (or gain) can be reduced to a simple equation: calories in/calories out.

That idea was the brainchild of two doctors, L.H. Newburgh and M.W. Johnston, at the University of Michigan. Their theory was an outgrowth of 'the body as a machine' thesis of many scientists of the time. Put simply, the doctors argued that if we consume fewer calories than our body burns, we are bound to lose weight. So if, for example, a body burns 2,500 calories in a day and its owner consumes only 1,500, this will lead to a 1,000-calorie deficit, which the body makes up for by burning stored fuel (fat). If we keep burning stored fuel to make up for this energy deficit, the result will be weight loss.

Doctors have been singing this tune for 80 years. In all that time there has not been any long-term scientific evidence to show that dieting is effective for long-term weight loss. And in all that time the population as a whole has been getting progressively heavier. At the last count around 64 per cent of the US population and 46 per cent of the European Union's population were obese. By 2007 this figure was expected to reach 68 and 48 per cent respectively.

If weight loss was simply a matter of cutting calories and being more active, then our population should be in pretty good shape. At any given time as much as 50 per cent of the population in the UK and elsewhere in the developed world is on a diet and/or an exercise regime. But we are not getting thinner.

Over and over again surveys like the one at UCLA show that the majority of people who lose weight on a given diet will subsequently regain that lost weight (and more besides). There is even evidence to suggest that dietary regimes that severely restrict calories, as well as specific types of foods (fats, carbohydrates and so on), are not terribly effective in the short term[8] and actually encourage rebound weight gain over the longer term.[9]

This rebound effect, which is well known to dieters, is also well documented in medical literature. Nutritionists believe that it may have deep roots in human evolution. In our hunter-gatherer stage, when the next meal was unpredictable, we became programmed to overeat when food was abundant. In times of food deprivation (including when we diet), our ancient hard-wiring kicks in. Our bodies employ mechanisms, largely driven by hormones, to store calories by overriding signals of satiety (fullness and satisfaction) and increasing hunger signals, even when food becomes plentiful again. In essence, the body is storing up calories in anticipation of the next period of food deprivation – even if it never comes.

According to the data, this effect is more dramatic when food and drink are freely available, when the available foods are calorie-dense (such as crisps, carbonated drinks, hamburgers and 'healthy' cereal bars) and when energy expenditure is low, due to reduced physical activity.

Medical science has determined a biological basis for this storage effect. The speed at which the body burns fuel is known as its 'metabolism'. When we lose weight, our basal metabolic rate (BMR) – the minimum amount of energy that the body requires at rest, to keep the body alive and to maintain weight at a constant 'set point' – decreases. BMR is related to the actual amount of body tissue, so it naturally decreases when the amount of body tissue is reduced through dieting.

Dieters who have been brought up on the calories in/calories out philosophy may still believe that skipping meals and going hungry is the best way to lose weight. But skipped meals mean that the body is more likely to store subsequent meals as fat. When calories are restricted, the body – which is an intelligent living system – recognizes that food is in short supply and does its best to conserve any existing stores of energy. In effect, it adapts itself to the reduced supply and starts to burn progressively less fat.

Indeed, in one animal study, rats were examined as they were put through several cycles of weight gain and weight loss. Each time these animals lost and regained weight, their metabolism progressively slowed – so much so that the weight loss in the second cycle was half as fast as it was in the first, and the weight came back three times as quickly.[10] This effect has also been confirmed in humans.[11]

The rebound effect may be particularly dangerous in child dieters, setting up a lifetime of almost uncontrollable weight. Studies show that dieting in pre-adolescents and adolescents results in excess weight gain over time.[12] In a recent large-scale study involving more than 15,000 children (aged 9–14 years), followed over a three-year period, it was found that dieters gained significantly more weight than matched non-dieters.[13] The authors concluded that self-directed dieting in this age group was not only ineffective, but actually promoted weight gain.

Constant yo-yoing of weight through dieting and bingeing plays havoc with the body's BMR and set point, in some cases wiping out the set point altogether, leaving the body with no blueprint for maintaining a healthy weight.

Severe calorie restriction forces the body to use not only fat, to make up for the energy deficit, but protein as well. The protein that the body uses as a top-up fuel comes from muscle. Muscle is metabolically demanding; essentially it is the body's engine room, where the bulk of the body's fuel is burned. When the body loses muscle bulk, its overall capacity to burn fuel declines as well. With this comes an inevitable decline in a person's ability to lose weight, and an increased likelihood that he or she will put weight on instead.

Fad diets are bad diets

Efficient metabolism is dependent on the supply of certain nutrients, such as magnesium and the B vitamins found in good quantities in whole grains. But during a diet it is not just food quantity, but also food *quality* that generally declines. With this decline there is almost an inevitable reduction in our intake of nutrients.

A combination of media-fuelled fads and bad nutritional advice is spurring dieters throughout the developed world to voluntarily (and unwisely) cut out healthy foods, and sometimes entire food groups, from their diets. In one 1999 survey by Gallup in the US, 32 per cent of dieters completely eliminated entire food groups when trying to lose weight.[14]

Twenty-eight per cent of those who took part in the survey eliminated all grains when dieting, but only 24 per cent eliminated fatty foods; 15 per cent cut out salty snacks; 15 per cent eradicated meat; and 13 per cent cut out dairy products. Only sweets were considered a greater threat to the waistline than grains.

For efficient fat-burning potential it is important to eat a wide variety of foods to keep up our intake of a range of essential nutrients.

The diet industry

In spite of the failure of conventional diets, the comforting equation of calories in/calories out still informs most weight-loss initiatives, possibly because it makes the job of 'doing something about it' so effortless. Weight-management programmes centred on this simple equation are easy to devise – anyone with a calculator, a calorie reference guide and an exercise manual can do it – and shift the responsibility for the success or failure of the regime squarely onto the individual.

It's a familiar scenario. When faced with difficult cultural problems, where challenging the status quo could raise uncomfortable questions, we tend to simplify. Consider the way that individuals are encouraged to switch off standby electronic items and change to energy-efficient light bulbs in order to 'do something' about climate change. Focusing on individual efforts – and failures – in this way deflects our attention away from bigger and arguably more powerful influences, such as the government subsidies that keep polluting airlines and industries in business.

Much the same is true of the food we eat. Food producers and manufacturers and pharmaceutical companies have enormous lobbying power. They have the power to define illness[15] and dictate policy and to influence where the blame gets placed when poorly thought-out health initiatives fail.

The way that we associate dieting with health and well-being, and even with beauty and attractiveness, effectively obscures the fact that the diet industry is a big and ruthless business. It has one goal: through diet foods, supplements, pills, exercise equipment, gyms, weight-loss clubs and magazines, it aims to convert sporadic dieters into permanent dieters, thereby increasing what we spend each year on trying to lose weight. The diet industry relies on the fact that vanity is no longer a vice, but a virtue; as well as relying on our infatuation with the quick fix – preferably one we can buy off the shelf.

So we spend to get thin; an estimated $48 billion on diet food and merchandise in the US – a figure that is forecast to reach $61 billion by 2008.[16] In the European Union we spend around 93 billion euros on diet products each year,[17] and the figure is growing.

The dieting industry, like much of modern medicine, is founded on the expectation of failure. Like the cigarette industry, the end product fosters its own demand. In this respect it has accepted the limitations of its own philosophy much more conclusively than the rest of us have. When God gives you lemons, as the saying goes, make lemonade. The high failure rate of diets makes for a lot of repeat business and a healthy bottom line. So health clubs, diet groups and slimming products are deeply dependent on the around 95 per cent of dieters for whom permanent weight loss is elusive.

The diet industry is, perhaps not surprisingly, an outgrowth of the pharmaceutical industry, and as such its reach is long.

Pharmaceutical companies are, for instance, the major sources of funding for obesity research, obesity groups and think tanks. They seed these particular fields, not in the name of science or public interest, but in the name of marketing. For example, in the US the 'consumer' group known as the American Obesity Association (which, by definition, should be giving out impartial advice) is largely funded by weight-loss companies, including Weight Watchers, Jenny Craig, Hoffman-La Roche and Slim-Fast.

To comprehend how this kind of funding can distort our understanding of weight and health, consider this: In June 1998 the National Institutes of Health (NIH) in the US asked 24 experts to write guidelines for diagnosing and treating obesity. The expert panel decided that obesity should be defined as a BMI of 30 or higher, and overweight as a BMI above 25 and below 30 (see box on pages 26–27).[18]

Before that time, an average woman – with a height of 1.6 m (5 ft 4 in), weighing 70 kg (155 lb) – was considered overweight; under the new guidelines, the definition of overweight dropped to 66 kg (145 lb). Similarly someone who is 1.8 m (5 ft 10 in) tall and weighs 83 kg (185 lb) was considered overweight under the previous guidelines; but under the new guidelines for the same height, 79 kg (175 lb) is overweight and 94 kg (209 lb) is obese.

Essentially, with a stroke of the pen, 25 million people who were not considered obese one day became obese the next – and were considered appropriate for medical treatments, including prescribed weight-loss drugs. The panel, which included the pharmacologist who created the heart-damaging and deadly phen-fen diet-pill combo (which was withdrawn from the market in 1997 because of is lethal consequences), was heavily criticized for its ties to the drug and weight-loss industries.[19] But the decision to keep the new BMI figures remained unchanged.

When, in 2004, the US Centers for Disease Control (CDC) classified obesity as a stand-alone disease, the move was heavily supported by the diet industry, which knew that as a result the government and private insurance would cover the use of their products by desperate dieters and that they could further lobby for tax deductions for obesity treatments.

Such is the corrupting influence of the diet industry that some scientists are beginning to question whether the obesity epidemic is as out of control as the media would have us believe. Recent accusations that in 2004 the CDC deliberately overestimated 'official' figures of the number of deaths attributable to obesity by some 20 per cent – in order to justify the classification of obesity as a disease – have not helped quell the discontent.[20]

By 2005 it was clear that the CDC had not just miscalculated, but had grossly misled doctors, scientists, politicians and the public when it stated that 400,000 people a year in the US died because they were obese. In May 2005 a researcher at the CDC published new data in the *Journal of the American Medical Association*[21] showing that the actual number of people who died from obesity in the US was 112,000. A reanalysis of the original CDC data also revealed something even more interesting. The death rates for people who were overweight were actually lower than those for people of normal weight; in all there were 86,000 fewer deaths in the overweight group. It also became clear that the negative effects of being obese were confined to those at the extreme end of the scale – those with a BMI of 35 or more.

At the same time in the UK an analysis of obesity statistics for England by the Social Issues Research Centre (SIRC) indicated that widespread assumptions about 'exponential' rises in obesity and the 'epidemic' scale of the problem were not justified by the data. In particular, obesity was a problem much more associated with middle age and later life than it was with children and teenagers. The SIRC report also commented on the somewhat arbitrary nature of the definition of obesity in childhood, when rapid changes in height, weight and body shape occur.[22]

These findings fuelled a rebound effect of their own. In a well-researched book entitled *Fat Politics – The Real Story Behind America's Obesity Epidemic*,[23] Associate Professor in Political Science at the University of Chicago, Eric Oliver, suggested that the obesity epidemic is largely a myth promoted by the weight-loss industry and by diet doctors, and that it is time to stop making body weight an indicator of a person's health. He also suggested that it is our panic over our weight gain, rather than the weight itself, that is probably causing most harm – and there is probably some truth in this. It is our panic that causes us to rely too heavily on 'experts', who seem to change their minds every year about what is healthy and what is not; and that causes us to look for quick fixes and to skim the surface of what is really causing our weight gain.

Calculating BMI

The healthy weight range that you see on many diet charts is based on a measurement known as the Body Mass Index (BMI). This can be determined in three steps if you know your weight and height.

1 Work out your height in metres and multiply the figure by itself.
2 Measure your weight in kilograms.
3 Divide the weight by the height squared (that is, the answer to Q1.)

So if, for example, you are 1.6 m (5 ft 3 in) tall and weigh 65 kg (140 lb), the calculation would be: 1.6 x 1.6 = 2.56; 65 divided by 2.56 = a BMI of 25.39.

If your BMI is	You are considered
18.5 or less	Underweight
18.5–24.9	Normal
25.0–29.9	Overweight
30.0–39.9	Obese
40 or greater	Extremely obese

Researchers and doctors like the concept of BMI because it is a shorthand that enables them to use a single number to describe the fatness of both a woman who is 1.5 m (5 ft) and a man who is 1.8 m (6 ft). To the average man or woman, BMI is still an abstract term; worse, it is largely meaningless.

For instance, BMI is not applicable or appropriate for children, pregnant women, older people or anyone with a long-term health condition. Nor is it infallible. It is possible, for example, for a healthy, muscular athlete with very low body fat to be classified as obese using the BMI formula.

The folly of BMI is further illustrated by the fact that under current standards for what is 'overweight' and 'obese', Brad Pitt is technically 'overweight', while Arnold Schwarzenegger is 'obese'.

How dieting changes us

For the purposes of this book, it is assumed that overweight and obesity are a growing problem, even if the scale of the problem is much less than is generally assumed. The key question is whether dieting is the way to address that problem. By all accounts the answer is no.

Dieting may not give us permanent weight loss, but it does have a profound effect on us in other ways. The dieting culture that has sprung up in the developed world amounts to a form of social, political and psychological assault on our bodies and our minds.

If half of us are dieting at any one time, this process of restricting what we eat, trying to be 'good' and 'disciplined', and feeling dissatisfied with who we are and the way we look is potentially a powerful social force. We should not underestimate how this shapes who we are, how we behave and how healthy we are in the long run.

Dieting changes us in many profound ways. For example, it:

• Changes what we eat, exposing us to dieting foods such as synthetic sweeteners and synthetic fats, foods made from additives and synthetic nutrients, which are in themselves toxic.

• Denies our enjoyment of food, so that we eat quickly and often alone; food becomes less social and more shameful.

• Focuses us on restriction and discipline. As such, it encourages unhealthy psychological divisions within the self (the 'good' side of our personality denies the body food, while the 'bad' side indulges). It also fosters self-hatred and often deep dissatisfaction with ourselves.

• Encourages false hope and a false sense of security, especially with regard to diet products. There has been an explosion in diet foods and supplements in recent years, and yet there is very little proof of their effectiveness (and in many cases almost no proof of safety). Surveys show that most of us assume that warnings are required on such products – this is not the case. Likewise, most of us believe that if a product is being sold in a shop, it has already been tested for safety – again, this is not the case.

• Leads to disordered eating, especially in adolescents. Teenage dieting is the usual antecedent to anorexia and bulimia nervosa. In prospective studies,[24] dieting has been associated with a fivefold to eighteenfold increased risk of developing an eating disorder. However, it is unclear whether dieting causes, triggers or represents the first stage to the illness. Several studies have documented the risk of binge-eating among dieting teenagers,[25] and a review of the psychological consequences of food deprivation in adults concluded that deprivation resulted in a tendency to overeat and even in binge-eating.[26]

• Promotes chronic illness. Continual dieting can lead to nutritional deficiencies, particularly of iron and calcium. These can also pose short- and long-term risks. In growing children and teenagers, for instance, even a marginal reduction in energy intake can be associated with poor growth.[27] Disordered eating, even in the absence of substantial weight loss, has been found to be associated with menstrual irregularities.[28] Over the longer term this can raise the risk of bone diseases such as osteopenia (mild thinning of the bone mass) and osteoporosis.[29] Because many very low-calorie diets include little fibre, constipation can be a problem. Chronic dieting also raises your risk of gallstones, liver dysfunction, protein, fluid and electrolyte imbalance and hair loss.

Drive carefully when dieting

If you are severely restricting your intake of calories to lose weight, you may end up being a danger to yourself and others. One 1997 study by a group of US and UK government scientists cut the number of calories in a small group of women by half for more than five months. Using standardized tests, the researchers found that the women's reaction times were slowed by an average of 6 per cent while on the calorie-restricted diet. What is more, the decline continued even after the women returned to eating their usual number of calories, reaching almost 11 per cent.[30]

The researchers expressed concern that the slowed reaction time could be enough to increase the risk of accidents, especially while driving. Perhaps, like some medications, very low-calorie diets should come with a warning: 'May decrease reaction time. Use care when operating a car or dangerous machinery.'

Rethinking fat

If the idea that diets don't work is difficult to accept, then the concept that fat is more than an unsightly storehouse for unused calories may be even more shocking. But again the research is clear.[31] Body fat is a vital organ, like your liver or kidneys, and its function is just as intricate as that of any other organ in the body.

Data suggests that body fat is biochemically sophisticated and complex. It responds to the body's needs, it produces vital hormones and it is much more crucial to our total health and well-being than was previously thought. It plays an important role in protecting bones and organs, regulating hormones and the immune system, and managing women's reproductive systems. It interacts with the nervous system, sending messages out to the body, such as when it's time to eat and when the body has had enough to eat. Its distribution around the body is responsive to outside or environmental influences, as well as to the presence of disease.[32]

One of the reasons why low-calorie diets don't work is because they are an extension of our simplistic view of fat: that it is simply an energy source to be used up. By denying the body essential calories, low-calorie diets take a rather mechanistic view of fat – that, through willpower, the body can be forced to burn away this stored energy to become 'healthy'. In fact, everything we know about fat suggests that before you lose it, you should try to understand it. And, as with all our other vital organs, we abuse our body fat at our peril.

Where fat goes

Studies comparing fat distribution in humans with that of other mammals show that even the leanest wild animals have fat on their bodies. Years ago an extraordinary investigation in the *New York Times*, based around the work of several eminent scientists, revealed the fate and purpose of fat in our bodies.[33] In both humans and other animals, fat tends to collect in similar locations around the body: on the breasts, the upper arms (or front legs in animals), around the tailbone and thighs, the abdomen and at the back of the neck. Because we need fat on our bodies to support us through lean times, the body will hold on to fat for handy energy, easily creating new fat cells and converting any fat in the diet into stores against a future famine.

The problem is that fat cells are also for ever. They can shrink or expand by up to ten times their original size, but they can never be destroyed. What is more, they can multiply. If, for instance, the amount of fat in the diet is too great for the existing number of fat cells to deal with, the body will produce new ones, and these also stay with you for ever.

But the *where* and *how* of fat is not nearly as interesting as the *why*. Fat does not get deposited around the body in a random fashion; wherever fat accumulates, it does so with a specific purpose. Thus, at some sites, fat deposits are better at absorbing fat molecules (lipids) from the bloodstream, while other deposits are better at releasing lipids to neighbouring tissue to be used as fast fuel.

For example, in many mammals, significant deposits of fat can be found naturally around the heart muscle – a discovery that has caused scientists to rethink the idea that fat around the heart is a dangerous pathological condition, caused solely by the high-fat Western diet. This fat around the heart has a dual purpose: it acts as a filter protecting the heart from receiving too much fat after an especially high-fat meal; but it can also respond to the heart's energy needs by diverting quick energy to heart muscle.

Further research has shown that fat around the abdomen (most common in men) is particularly responsive to stress hormones like adrenaline and cortisol. Triggered by these 'fight-or-flight' hormones, the fat cells also release fuel to the muscles and heart for quick action (see also pages 146–149).

Fat deposits around the thighs – the bane of so many women's lives – are extraordinarily efficient at absorbing fatty molecules from the bloodstream. If you eat a high-fat meal, it is the fat around your thighs that will help remove excess fat from your bloodstream quickly.

By contrast, the small deposits of fat that can be found between muscles are very efficient at soaking up glucose from the blood, thus helping to maintain a healthy blood-sugar balance. This in turn is released as fuel, as and when the muscles require it.

In a nutshell, by removing and redirecting fat in your food to storage sites like the thighs and abdomen, the body is acting in an intelligent way to protect and preserve itself. We all need fat in our diet and, as long as levels of fat remain within reason, the body is able to metabolize and store it as necessary. As levels of dietary fat in the diet rise, or as other influences such as fad or starvation diets or some of the other factors outlined in this book come into play, this intelligent system can become overwhelmed and may begin to malfunction.

Looking at leptin

Apart from its intelligent distribution around the body, the most intriguing aspect of fat is the role it plays in the regulation of weight. While we think of excess fat as the consequence of a body out of control, in many ways it can be seen as the body trying to regain control.

The concept of a biological factor in weight regulation is not new. The hypothalamus is a gland at the base of the brain that regulates eating patterns, body temperature and metabolism. Scientists have long understood this, but were not sure how the hypothalamus received information concerning the amount of fat that a person had in store.

The discovery of a hormone called leptin 12 years ago at the Rockefeller Institute in New York ushered in a new age of enlightenment and changed the entire map of our understanding of fat and obesity. In the intervening years, as studies have poured in, it has become apparent that leptin could be playing a far more important role in health than, for instance, cholesterol. However, few doctors are taught to pay attention to it, or even know much about the way it influences health and disease.

Leptin is a hormone involved in the long-term regulation of body weight.[34] While some cells in the gut and placenta also make small amounts of it, leptin is mainly produced by fat cells. It circulates in the blood and interacts on different tissues and organs, including skeletal muscle, the liver and the hypothalamus.

Leptin is the way that your fat stores speak to your brain. The messages it carries tell the body when to decrease energy intake and increase energy expenditure. They let your brain know when you are full, how much energy is available and, very importantly, what to do with it. It has a role to play in controlling lipid distribution, directing the body to store fat in fat cells rather than in, say, the liver, where fat deposits are linked to disorders such as diabetes.

The level of circulating leptin in the body appears to correspond to the amount of fat in the body. More body fat equals more circulating leptin. Conversely, as you diet, leptin levels decline. But although overweight and obese people have a higher amount of leptin in their bodies, they seem to become increasingly insensitive to its signals. What is not yet clear is whether or not obesity causes a resistance to leptin, or vice versa.

As with all hormones, we need the right amount of leptin at the right times in our development in order to be healthy. Studies have shown that the correct balance of leptin – and the body's ability to respond to it – plays a significant (if not primary) role in heart disease, obesity, diabetes, osteoporosis, autoimmune diseases, reproductive disorders and perhaps the rate of ageing itself. Animal research, for instance, suggests that leptin surges shortly after birth are responsible for the correct development of those parts of the brain that control food intake and maintain a steady weight.[35]

Other research suggests that leptin may also be the missing link between obesity and diabetes. A 2005 animal study in the journal *Cell Metabolism* suggested that it regulates blood sugar through two different brain-body pathways: one that controls appetite and fat storage, and another that tells the liver what to do with its glucose reserves.[36] While animal research is not always directly conclusive in humans, studying leptin in humans can be difficult, since it requires a brain biopsy – something for which few human trial participants will volunteer.

It is already known that disrupting leptin's appetite-controlling role leads to obesity, and that obesity is known to significantly raise the risk of diabetes. But the data from the 2005 study suggests that it may take disruptions to both pathways to bring on full-blown diabetes and overwhelm the body's ability to control blood-glucose levels via the action of insulin.

Leptin has also been implicated in immune-system functioning and the development of bones. And it plays a role in reproductive function, regulating the onset of puberty in women. Individuals who are deficient in leptin tend to mature sexually at a slower rate, and this could be related to the amount of fat that is stored.

Scientists speculate that the many, seemingly unrelated effects of leptin may have evolved to enable animals to adapt to starvation. These days, the challenge in developed societies is to remain lean during times of abundance: obesity and diabetes are far more threatening than starvation. Indeed, studies into the role of leptin have served to emphasize why it is sometimes so hard to lose weight. Essentially, from an evolutionary perspective, we were built to store energy (fat), and we were programmed not to starve to death.

Scientists are currently speculating that leptin could be synthesized and made into a drug that can treat obesity – effectively tricking the brain into believing the body is full. Some animal studies have shown promising results. But to date no human studies have successfully proven this theory, and this has reinforced the belief that in obese individuals some kind of leptin resistance develops over time.

The folly of interfering with hormone levels in the body – for instance, with birth-control pills or HRT – should by now be obvious. Leptin is no exception. In 2007 a team at the University of California, San Diego, found that leptin triggered increased growth in human colon-cancer cells. The study published in the *British Journal of Surgery* could help to explain why severely overweight people, whose fat cells naturally produce more leptin in an attempt to regain metabolic balance, appear to be at far greater risk of the disease.[37]

The results of that study were a good illustration of the fact that you can get too much of a good thing. It is also a statement about how our bodies cannot be divided into 'stand-alone' chemicals and tissues. The way the body works is rather like an orchestra, and good health is the result of all the players working in harmony. As the next chapter shows, simplistic diet plans and pills that attack one aspect of the metabolism without considering all the others will never work in the complex orchestra of the human body, as well as in the complex modern environment in which it lives.

CHAPTER 2

The bigger picture

When faced with the idea that weight gain and weight loss are complex processes, proponents of the 'calories in/calories out' school of thinking start to get nervous. Their main objection to this view is that any acknowledgement of that complexity gives 'fat people' (and the presumption is always that this is a homogenous group) an 'excuse' to be 'lazy' and 'undisciplined'.

So before we go any further, let's clearly address some of that anxiety. What you eat, and how active you are, are influential on how much you weigh. If you spend your life sitting in front of the television sucking down burgers and beer, and if the only exercise you get is the trip to the fridge, you will become fat. Indeed, that sort of lifestyle will probably kill you.

What this book is attempting to do is to broaden your understanding of the co-factors that make weight gain more likely and weight loss more difficult. Whenever we broaden our understanding of a complex subject, it inevitably undermines the quick-fix mentality that has become a mainstay of so much of modern life.

The chances are that if you have picked up this book, it is probably because you are already aware that the quick fix does not work. Maybe you have tried eating properly, have tried low-calorie diets, have tried joining a gym and have seen few or no permanent results from your efforts. You want to lose weight, but weight loss is eluding you. The reason? Weight loss has little to do with willpower. It is information you need, not willpower. Having this information can, eventually, be liberating – but when we first recognize the complexity of life, and the human body, it can also be frustrating. After all, if fad diets and diet products don't work, and simply counting calories isn't enough, what are you to do?

There is probably no point in asking your doctor to answer that question. Most doctors have not yet made the conceptual changes necessary to see the bigger picture concerning what contributes to the increasing problem of overweight and obesity. And yet medical literature is replete with studies that illuminate and greatly extend our knowledge of the factors that contribute to weight gain and weight loss.

What we know and what we don't know are changing daily, but before embarking mindlessly on yet another low-calorie diet that may end in disappointment, it is worth considering the multitude of influences on the body's natural weight-management systems.

The usual suspects

A raft of scientific and medical data shows that weight gain is a multifactorial problem related to lifestyle and environment, and not simply to calories consumed. Where you live, what your income is, your level of education and your family history all play a part in determining not just your weight, but also your general level of health and well-being. Genetics may also play a part – though our understanding of how big or small that contribution is remains incomplete.

Most intriguingly, the kinds of everyday pollutants that you are exposed to, either at work or at home, may trigger weight gain in a much more significant way than could ever have been predicted at the end of the Second World War, when we effectively became a chemical society. It's worth taking a closer look at each of these factors in turn.

The urban lifestyle

Looked at from a global perspective, it is impossible not to acknowledge the multifaceted and devastating impact that urbanization and industrialization have had on our health. They have altered what we eat, when we eat, how much we eat, how often we eat and the quality of the food we eat, as well as our levels of daily physical exertion. In the developed world, urbanization has changed our lives beyond recognition – and not always for the better.

Because of urbanization and modernization, our lives are becoming more sedentary than ever before. Urbanization has ushered in profound changes in work patterns, lifestyles, family structures and value systems. These changes have had a knock-on effect on dietary practices and on our levels of physical activity. The urban lifestyle has become so much a part of who we are that we are barely able to see the way it affects the various aspects of our lives, including our weight. But in developing nations the startling parallel between the rise in obesity and the rapid acceptance of urban/industrial lifestyles and diets is all too apparent.

In many developing countries, the increasing mechanization of jobs and transportation, the greater availability of processed and fast foods and the growing dependence on television for leisure mean that people are swiftly adopting less physically active lifestyles and consuming more high-calorie, low-nutrient diets.[1]

Speaking at the International Congress on Obesity in Sydney in September 2006, Dr Philip James, the British chairman of the International Obesity Task Force (IOTF), noted that in China the rate of obesity has risen from almost zero in the 1980s to about 10 per cent of the population in 2006. That rise, he said, can be pinned down to the growing problems of urbanization and the infiltration of a generally nutritionally poor Western diet, which favours high-fat, high-energy products over basic fruits and vegetables.[2] Hong Kong is likewise facing a childhood obesity crisis, with the percentage of overweight schoolchildren in Hong Kong almost doubling in the past 13 years[3] – less than half a generation – and similar increases have been noted amongst more affluent urban dwellers in India.[4]

Junk food

The growing popularity of fast food is just one of many cultural changes that have been brought about by globalization.[5] Of the two perceived culprits – junk food and lack of exercise – it is the presence of the former in our diets that is perhaps the more pervasive, and persuasive, in terms of difficult-to-control weight gain.

According to a report by Harvard researchers in 2004, cheap convenience foods have become the main driving force behind rising rates of obesity in the West. Based in part on food diaries kept by the study's participants, a surprising picture of American eating habits emerged. In the US, people are not consuming any more calories at mealtimes than they did 20 years ago, but they have nearly doubled their consumption of calories from small snacks and carbonated drinks between meals.

The greater availability of snack foods is largely the result of waste and overproduction. Food companies, seeking an outlet for the glut of cereals and other raw foodstuffs in the 1980s and 1990s, developed literally hundreds of new products that increased the demand for food beyond previously imagined levels. The industry also took advantage of the burgeoning science of chemical flavouring and new technologies for processing and preserving foods to create high-fat, high-sugar and high-taste foods, and within just a few years processed foods became cheaper, more convenient and, importantly, tastier.

At the same time snacking was legitimized, as American culture celebrated the practice of 'grazing' – having several small meals throughout the day – as a supposedly healthy alternative to the more conventional three-meals-a-day approach.

Some people might reason that the convenience and pleasure of snack foods are worth carrying a few extra pounds for, but obesity carries with it a higher risk of developing type-2 diabetes, hypertension (high blood pressure), heart disease and other serious illnesses.

Although the study was conducted in the US, the results could easily have come from Britain or Australia, or from anywhere else where the free market rules the food industry, where regulatory systems are lax and allow almost any number of additives to be put in foods, and where snacking on junk foods (and, as a result, obesity) is on the rise.

Exercise

Exercise has many benefits in terms of keeping bones and muscles healthy and toned. Regular exercise also has a profound influence on our feelings of well-being. But the influence of exercise on overall weight loss is not at all clear-cut. Several large studies have recently shown, for instance, that increasing your level of physical activity is unlikely, on its own, to cause a substantial loss of weight.

In a 2006 Glasgow University study, published in the *British Medical Journal*, increasing activity amongst more than 500 four-year-olds, by adding three extra half-hour sessions of physical play and activity every week, made no difference to the children's weight.[6] Similar results have been found in adults.[7] Such results have perplexed researchers, but may, in part, have something to do with the rather simplistic maths that we apply to exercise when it comes to the calories in/calories out equation.

In September 2006, Ralph La Forge, managing director of the Duke Lipid and Disease Management Preceptorship Program at Duke University Medical Center, in North Carolina, compiled a detailed analysis of the various factors that influence the effect of exercise on weight loss.[8]

He began by refuting the long-held belief that since a pound (454 g) of fat (when burned) gives off 3,500 calories, and since walking briskly for a mile (1.6 km) burns 100 calories, a person should lose a pound for every 35 miles (56 km). In other words, all other things being equal, if a previously sedentary person starts running or walking 5 miles (8 km) a day, that person should lose a pound a week.

The problem with this estimate is that it fails to subtract the number of calories that the person's body would have used anyway, had it just sat still for the same amount of time. To calculate the actual number of calories you will lose each day, you must first subtract the number of calories burned by the old activity from the number of calories burned by the new activity.

So, for example, someone weighing 70 kg (154 lb) would burn 70 calories per hour just sitting still. This would need to be subtracted from the total calories burned in any other exercise, in order to burn more calories per hour.

Furthermore, if you walk or run on a treadmill, the aid of the machine diminishes the number of calories that your body uses, by about 10–15 per cent of what the machine says you are burning. So you have to run longer and faster to get the same results.

Your starting weight is also a factor: if you weigh less than 70 kg (154 lb), the caloric burn is proportionately less; if you weigh more than that, it is higher (see chart below).

This doesn't mean that exercise is not important. When you diet without exercising, you lose both muscle *and* fat. This is counterproductive, because muscle tissue is very metabolically active. With muscle wastage, your body's basic metabolic rate – that is, the number of calories that your body uses at rest – becomes slower.

Burning calories per hour			
Activity	54 kg (120 lb)	70 kg (154 lb)	77 kg (170 lb)
Aerobic dance	354	422	518
Basketball	330	440	460
Bicycling (indoor, hard effort)	572	733	810
Bicycling (outdoor, under 16 kph/10 mph)	236	281	345
Bowling	165	210	230
Callisthenics (light)	266	317	388
Cleaning	207	246	302
Eating (sitting)	80	105	115
Gardening	275	330	385
Golf (walking)	250	330	345
Hiking	330	370	460
Horseriding	220	279	310
Mowing lawn	300	384	425

Racquetball	385	489	540
Reading	70	91	100
Rowing (stationary)	385	489	540
Running (16 kph/10 mph)	880	1,118	1,230
Sitting (watching TV)	55	70	75
Sitting (writing, typing)	100	105	140
Skating, roller	385	489	540
Skiing, cross-country	440	559	615
Skiing, downhill	385	419	540
Swimming (leisure)	330	419	460
Tennis	375	489	540
Walking (brisk)	220	265	310
Water aerobics	218	279	308
Weight training (light)	165	220	230
Yoga (Hatha)	136	175	193

Note: these are general estimates; the actual amount you burn per activity per hour may vary with sex, age, weight and height.

Social class

In the developed world we like to think there is no class structure. But this is, of course, incorrect. Politicians don't like to talk about it, doctors and scientists don't always take it into account in their diagnoses and calculations, but poverty and disadvantage have a marked influence on the rise in obesity. Indeed, for some social classes they can be more influential than either food intake or exercise. Once considered a problem related to affluence, obesity is now fast-growing in many developing countries and in impoverished neighbourhoods of the developed world.[9]

The data shows quite clearly that lower-income families and those living in socially deprived neighbourhoods are far more at risk of becoming obese than those in the middle and upper classes.[10] For example, a report from the National Statistics office states:

> *Obesity is linked to social class, being more common among those in the routine or semi-routine occupational groups than the managerial and professional groups. The link is stronger among women. In 2001, 30 per cent of women in routine occupations were classified as obese compared with 16 per cent in higher managerial and professional occupations.*[11]

Researchers at the Department of Social Medicine at Bristol University have also found an association between deprivation and childhood obesity. Their 2004 study of more than 20,000 English children, aged between five and 14 years, concluded that:

> *... social origins may have a long term impact on obesity. Whether this operates through the early establishment of behavioural patterns, such as diet and exercise, or through metabolic changes associated with early deprivation, is still to be determined.*[12]

The authors of the Bristol study did not delve deeply into how social class affected weight gain, although it is apparent that relative deprivation affects not only levels of childhood obesity, but – and perhaps even more so – obesity in later adulthood.

Other research evidence suggests a direct link between obesity and poverty. In less privileged social classes, for example, obesity is more of a problem for women and young girls.

In the UK, for instance, the prevalence of obesity amongst women is only around 14 per cent in the highest social class, whereas in the lowest social class, double that number are obese.[13] Higher-than-average levels of obesity have also been found amongst some minority ethnic groups. In the 16–34 age group, 19.5 per cent of black Caribbean and 15 per cent of Pakistani young women are obese, compared with 12.7 per cent of women of the same age in the general population.[14]

Studies suggest that the lower the income, the higher the tendency towards a fast-food diet with little nutritional value. In lower-income groups there is also a higher rate of smoking and alcohol consumption, both of which are linked to a less healthy lifestyle that includes poor food choices and lack of exercise.

Thus, amongst the less affluent members of society, obesity and overweight are not really a medical problem, but a social one. It may not simply be that people on lower incomes don't know how to eat well. Instead, it may be that they do not know, or have forgotten, how to shop well. Likewise, in lower-income neighbourhoods, access to fresh food may be restricted. If you live in a tower block, where the only shop close to you is a convenience store selling a high proportion of snack foods and pre-packed meals, making healthy food choices is nearly impossible.

There is also a lingering perception that fresh foods are more expensive than convenience foods. And that making a meal from scratch is a thankless, time-consuming task. Worse, there is a belief that if a particular food is advertised on television or is on sale in a shop, then it can't be that bad for you.

Apart from providing lower-income families with the means to live more healthily, perhaps governments could be making inroads into showing people how to choose the building blocks of a better diet, or into making sure that farmers' markets find subsidized spaces in more impoverished neighbourhoods, so that everyone has access to fresh healthy, natural foods.

Genetic inheritance

Our genes are both the building blocks and blueprint for the way we look, the way we behave, the way our bodies function and our inherent biological strengths and weaknesses. For years we have laboured under the impression that all humans have the same genetic make-up. Those who deviate in some way from this basic blueprint are the ones, say scientists, who will be more prone to illness, disease or aberrations in behaviour.

The Human Genome Project, which was a 13-year project coordinated by the US Department of Energy and the National Institutes of Health, sought to unlock the secrets of the genetic influence on human health and disease by identifying and studying all the approximately 20,000–25,000 genes in human DNA. Clearly some genetic deviations do produce illness and some of these – for instance, haemophilia, cystic fibrosis, Huntington's disease and sickle-cell disease – can be very serious. However, one of the most interesting findings of the human genome project is that there are no genetically 'pure' types. We are all unique; we all deviate from previously perceived norms in some way.[15] As this has become apparent, scientists have been forced to reassess the real impact of genetics on health and disease.

The deeper we look into this issue, the more it becomes apparent that genetic inheritance plays only a minor role in many of the diseases that we associate with modern life or with ageing.

For instance, our genes have very little to do with how we age or how long we live.[16] Similarly, for autoimmune diseases such as arthritis, environmental factors may be more important than genetics.[17] New evidence also suggests that for many years studies estimating the lifetime risk of women with the BRCA1 and BRCA2 genetic mutation developing breast cancer, or getting recurring breast cancer, have overestimated that risk by nearly

100 per cent.[18] Other factors, say scientists, such as lifestyle and environment, are more influential.

The same is true for being overweight. So although we often say being overweight is 'in our genes', it probably isn't – at least not to the extent that we hope.

Nevertheless, as the obesity problem gets worse, scientists have gone into overdrive to try and find a genetic explanation for why people seem to be getting fatter, even though our diets – at least for some – appear to be getting better. For years the search has focused on finding an obesity gene.

Scientific study can show to a limited extent how individual genes influence weight gain. But no full picture has emerged on what might trigger an obesity gene to make us fat, or how it can be manipulated to make us thin. Indeed, scientists are currently investigating some 250 genes that they believe are linked to obesity, and although the results are often trumpeted in the news, the reality is rather less impressive.

GAD2 In 2003 research by scientists at Imperial College, London, suggested that the GAD2 gene causes production of a chemical – gamma-amino butyric acid – that increases a person's appetite. The finding was widely heralded as a breakthrough. But in their report, published in the *Public Library of Science Biology*, the scientists cautioned that although their research is significant, obesity cannot be explained by a single factor.[19] Two years later a different group of scientists, writing in the same journal, were unable to reproduce the findings of the first study.[20]

Ob While some recent news stories have referred to this gene as '*the* obesity gene', the truth is rather less impressive. The Ob gene is responsible for obesity in one strain of mice. To date, no more than five human beings on the planet, who have been identified with a mutation in this gene, are known to be obese as a result of having the Ob gene. What this means is that, although variations or mutations in this gene may be responsible for a very small number of extreme cases of obesity, it probably does not play a substantial role in most cases of human obesity.

Lep-R Once known as the db (diabetes) gene, Lep-R also leads to obesity in a particular strain of mice. This gene helps to make the body receptive to the effects of leptin (see page 32), signalling a feeling of satiety. A few individuals do have mutations or variations in the Lep-R gene that make them unusually insensitive to leptin, but these are extraordinarily rare cases.

B$_3$ In August of 1995 three research papers appeared in the *New England Journal of Medicine* describing the B$_3$ gene.[21] Although variations in this gene appear to have some interesting associations with aspects of diabetes and metabolism, the evidence of any relation to body weight or body fatness was, at best, extremely weak.

FTO In 2007 researchers announced the discovery of what they believed was the first and clearest common genetic link to obesity yet found. They reviewed data on more than 38,000 children and adults in the UK and Europe, looking for a genetic anomaly that would explain individual susceptibility to diabetes. By accident they found that a certain variation in the FTO gene was associated with extra body fat, obesity and type-2 diabetes.[22]

The strength of the genetic influence depends on whether an individual has inherited one or two copies of the FTO-gene variant. Thus someone with two copies of the FTO variant was likely, on average, to weigh 3 kg (6½ lb) more than someone who does not have the FTO variant at all, and if they have only one copy, they were likely to weigh 1.2 kg (2½ lb) more.

In this study one in six participants had two copies of the FTO-gene variation, and these people were found to have an increased risk of obesity of approximately 67 per cent and of type-2 diabetes of about 40 per cent.

It seemed like an important result, but an extra 1.2–3 kg (2½–6½ lb) in weight does not make a person obese, and unfortunately the study did not examine the participants' diet and exercise habits. In the press furore that followed, the researchers admitted that they really don't know exactly how the FTO gene might affect body fat or weight.

There is some science to show that heredity and obesity are linked. In one Danish study, published in the *New England Journal of Medicine*, adults who were adopted as children were found to have weights closer to those of their biological parents than to those of their adoptive parents. In this case, a person's genetic make-up had more influence on the development of obesity than the environment in the adoptive family home.[23] Statistics show that a child with two obese parents has an 80 per cent risk of becoming overweight, while a child with just one obese parent has a 40 per cent risk, and a child with normal-weight parents has a 7 per cent risk of becoming overweight. This would suggest that, even if we cannot explain why, obesity tends to run in families, and such data is suggestive of a genetic cause.

But we all inherit much more than biology from our families. Families share diets and lifestyles, attitudes and habits, as well as a physical environment that may contribute to obesity. Separating these from genetic factors is often difficult. Indeed, the key to the unpredictable nature of genetic risk factors may lie in multifactorial triggers, like environment and lifestyle.

The truth is that there is always going to be someone who

believes that genetics holds the key to life's problems. In truth, genetics often raises more questions than it answers. Genetic susceptibility does not equal weight gain, just as genetic susceptibility does not equal cancer. Something has to push the genetic button for these minor variations in a person's make-up to become significant.

Mapping metabolism

We may be no closer to discovering a 'fat gene', but recent evidence from the University of California at Irvine suggests that some aspects of heredity do influence our dietary needs and the way our bodies metabolize food.[24] According to geneticist Douglas Wallace and his colleagues, mitochondrial deoxyribonucleic acid (DNA) is responsible for the body's adaptation to different climates. The mitochondria – the powerhouse of the human cell – generate energy by telling the body to eat.

After looking at differences in climate, researchers found that people in warmer climates have extremely efficient mitochondria, which use more energy for work than for producing heat. Less efficient mitochondria, such as those that people in colder climates possess, store more of the energy they receive from food to produce heat.

But this adaptive response might not be beneficial when people native to one climate relocate to another. For example, people who live in tropical or equatorial regions have a strong hereditary need for high-carbohydrate diets that are rich in vegetables, fruits, grains and legumes. These foods tend to provide the kind of body fuel that is most compatible with an active lifestyle in warm and humid regions of the world. Their systems are simply not designed to process or utilize large quantities of animal protein and fat.

Conversely, people from cold, harsh northern climates are not genetically equipped to survive on light vegetarian food. They tend to burn body fuel quickly, and so need heavier foods to sustain themselves. Inuit people living in their native climate, for example, can easily digest and assimilate large quantities of protein and fat – the very types of foods that would overwhelm the digestive tracts of people from the Mediterranean basin. Either way, a move from your native climate may end up causing lifelong weight gain and a host of other related illnesses.

Such evidence throws up more questions than it answers – for instance, what climate is best for those who are 'mixed' types, with no straightforward genetic heritage? From the perspective of the weather and health, however, it might explain why a cold snap in an otherwise moderate climate may cause such devastating health effects. Under such circumstances, the cells may simply not be able to adjust their heat-producing mechanism quickly enough.

The unusual suspects

The ongoing failure of gold-standard solutions such as calorie-counting has motivated some scientists to suggest that we must be missing something and to look beyond the usual explanations.

In 2006 a paper in the *International Journal of Obesity* courageously attempted to explore the 'roads less travelled' in obesity research, and suggested at least ten additional factors for obesity that have nothing to do with the usual sins of gluttony and sloth.[25]

The authors, made up of a panel of doctors from across the US, concluded that medical science had a tendency to 'focus overwhelmingly on food marketing practices and technology and on institution-driven reductions in physical activity (the "Big Two"), eschewing the importance of other influences'.

The panel went on to say that the influence of the Big Two on the global obesity epidemic is 'largely circumstantial', relying as it does on broad surveys rather than on epidemiological data focused on individuals or large randomized studies. They further noted that the acceptance of the idea that too much food and too little exercise is the sole cause of obesity '... has created a hegemony whereby the importance of the Big Two is accepted as established and other putative factors are not seriously explored. The results may be well intentioned, but ill-founded, proposals for reducing obesity.'

In an effort to broaden the debate, the authors suggested that since being overweight or obese was a modern problem, perhaps many of the putative contributors to the problem may also have their roots in modern life. And this was borne out by their comparative review of the available research. Their conclusion was that even if some of these causes have only a small effect, they may interact with each other and with other factors in ways that greatly magnify their individual effects.

The ten most prominent contributors to obesity and overweight in this particular review were:

1 Sleep debt. Too many of us are getting too little sleep and the resulting 'sleep debt' can alter hormone levels and trigger an increase in body weight. Sleep debt is also associated with insulin resistance and diabetes and with increased hunger and appetite.

2 Pollution. Hormones control body weight and many of today's pollutants drastically alter levels of key hormones. Significantly, many of these pollutants are lipophilic (fat-loving). Once in the body, they get stored in fat and, because they are so toxic, the body resists burning fat and thus liberating these toxins back into the bloodstream.

3 Air conditioning. We burn more calories when the environment is too hot or too cold for comfort. But more people than ever live and work in temperature-controlled homes and offices. This has lowered the number of calories that we burn each day.

4 Decreased smoking. Because of its effects on the circulation and the nervous system, smoking reduces weight. In many developed countries people are smoking much less than they used to. While no one would suggest taking up smoking as a means to lose weight in the 21st century, we will have to deal with the effects of first poisoning our bodies with tobacco (creating a false thinness) and then coming off the drug, which can cause a rebound (but temporary) weight gain.

5 Prescription medication. Many different drugs – including contraceptives, steroid hormones, diabetes drugs, some anti-depressants and blood-pressure drugs – can cause weight gain. Use of these drugs has risen exponentially in recent decades to combat other 21st-century diseases.

6 Population age and ethnicity. Middle-aged people and those of African, Hispanic and Pakistani origin have a tendency to be more obese than younger people of European descent. Throughout the world the population is getting older and more ethnically diverse.

7 Older mothers. The average age at which a woman has her first child is rising. There is some evidence that the older a woman is when she gives birth, the higher her child's risk of obesity.

8 Ancestry and environment. Some health problems are passed down through the generations. A tendency towards gestational diabetes will produce a child prone to obesity (who is in turn more likely to produce obese children). Very high-fat diets during pregnancy have been shown, in animals, to skew the metabolism of offspring two generations down the line.

9 Obesity linked to fertility. Some evidence suggests that overweight and obese people are more fertile than lean ones. If obesity does have a genetic component, that makes it a dominant characteristic, and the percentage of obese people in the population is likely to increase.

10 Like marrying like. Obese women tend to marry obese men. If there are fewer thin people around – and if obesity is a dominant genetic characteristic – then these couples will produce obese children, who will then go on to produce more obese children in the next generation.

Since the publication of that paper, other research has emerged suggesting links with excessive time spent watching television. Allergies and inflammation can also contribute to obesity.

You can't always 'do something' about these factors. Some (like heredity) are simply a part of you, but others (such as sleep debt and environmental pollutants) are within your control, and dealing with them may make a substantial contribution to helping you slim down. The next few chapters focus on those factors that you *can* do something about.

CHAPTER 3

Sleep yourself thin

The 'epidemic' of obesity in our society is paralleled by another less obvious, but equally disastrous epidemic: lack of sleep.

In our 'open all hours' culture it's easy to trivialize the role of sufficient sleep in staying healthy And yet nothing is more effective than a good night's sleep in maintaining a healthy body, mind and soul. Unfortunately, for many people sound, uninterrupted sleep remains an elusive goal; around one-third of us suffer from some type of sleep difficulty. Even those who don't are often short-changed when it comes to sleep: we work long hours, or are employed to work nights or shift work; we squeeze family commitments into the time that is left, and end up sacrificing sleep in order to fit it all in.

Research shows that as the years go by we are sleeping less and less. Thirty years ago adults slept for around seven and a half hours per night; 80 years ago they slept even longer, for around close to nine hours a night. Even though sleep professionals and other experts recommend eight hours of sleep per night, today – according to the US National Sleep Foundation – most adults only sleep an average of 6.85 hours per night.

For the first time, scientists are looking seriously at what happens to our bodies when we live on less sleep than we need and the health implications are shocking. Their conclusion is that sleep is like money in the bank: if you keep taking it out without putting any back in, you will eventually become bankrupt. A flood of new research now confirms that sleep is not (as is commonly believed) a passive state; it is a highly active and complex state that is vital to our physical, mental and emotional health.

Several key hormones are disrupted by lack of sleep. The normal daily rhythm of intense sunlight alternating with nights of near-total darkness has dominated the planet for many thousands of years. The artificial light that bombards city dwellers in particular can drastically alter this cycle. The attempt to erase the night (or at least limit it to small, artificially confined 'windows') may come at a high price. It can, at a minimum, lead to a chronic lack of sleep, diminishing the effectiveness of the body's immune system. But studies also show that it can disrupt levels of a hormone called melatonin, the knock-on effect of which can be an increased risk of certain cancers, such as breast cancer (see box on pages 72–73).

Sleep is also necessary for proper immune function and to help regulate the endocrine (hormone) system. Lack of sleep has long been known to impact on heart health,[1] mood and memory.[2]

Chronic sleep loss can also substantially affect weight control, reducing the body's ability to perform basic metabolic functions, such as processing and storing carbohydrates or regulating hormone secretion. So profound is the link that some scientists believe that lack of sleep may be one of the most important links between the triumvirate of chronic debilitating conditions – diabetes, hypertension and obesity – commonly grouped under the diagnostic umbrella of Metabolic Syndrome, or Syndrome X.

The greater your accumulated 'sleep debt', the greater the risk of suffering from a whole range of disorders, including hard-to-shift weight. Worse, once you have acquired a sleep debt, it can be hard to make it up again. Evidence suggests that even after four straight nights of uninterrupted quality sleep, deprived people are still slower and more prone to errors than those who have not lost any sleep.

Sleep debt and obesity

The amount of sleep we get each night is also important to hormone regulation. When we don't sleep long enough or well enough, levels of several important hormones (including those responsible for regulating body weight and metabolism) became disrupted. Other evidence shows that sleep debt decreases the brain's ability to function fully – most significantly, impairing those areas of the brain responsible for attention, complex planning, sophisticated mental operations and judgement. Nutritionists believe that this interference with 'executive function' – the ability to make clear, sound decisions – may also impact on how we choose to eat when we are awake.

The connection between lack of sleep and obesity has been demonstrated in large population studies across all age groups. Most recently a study at the University of Warwick found that sleep deprivation was associated with an almost twofold increase in the risk of being obese – for both children and adults.[3] The research reviewed the current evidence in more than 28,000 children and 15,000 adults and concluded that the less we sleep, the greater our risk of an increased BMI (see pages 26–27), a higher waist circumference and of becoming obese over time.

This risk was evident in children as young as five years old.

Yet another very large study in 2004 at Columbia University, New York, found that those who got less than four hours of sleep a night were 73 per cent more likely to be obese than those who got the recommended seven to nine hours. Those who averaged five hours of sleep had a 50 per cent greater risk, and those who got six hours a 23 per cent greater risk.[4]

In other recent research published in the *Archives of Internal Medicine* in 2005, US researchers from Eastern Virginia Medical School confirmed that weight went up as sleep time went down.[5] So strong was the evidence that the scientists made an urgent call for more research into the impact of incorporating better sleep into weight-loss regimes.

The editorial in the same edition of that journal broke with the tradition of sterile scientific language and pulled no punches, especially with regard to the implications of this research concerning increasing levels of childhood obesity:

It is now crucial to determine the importance of lack of sufficient sleep during the early formative years in putting our youth on a trajectory toward obesity and the metabolic syndrome – a trajectory that could be altered if sleep loss is indeed playing a role in this epidemic.

Other studies confirm these findings, in all age groups, even the very young:

• Using sleep data taken from more than one million adults in the US, a study by the American Cancer Society found that a relationship between short sleep duration and obesity was evident. This data also showed an association between sleep duration and early mortality.[6]

• In a sample of 496 Swiss adults followed up over 13 years, there was a steady increase in Body Mass Index (BMI) from 21.8 to 23.3 between the ages of 27 and 40 years, with a concurrent decrease in sleep duration from 7.1 to 6.9 hours a night in men, and from 7.7 to 7.3 hours in women. This study also noted that the association between short sleep duration and obesity diminished with age; therefore this association may be most important early on in life, when it may have the greatest impact on setting future eating habits.[7]

• In a Japanese study of 8,274 children, aged six to seven years, the odds of obesity were about three times greater for those sleeping less than eight hours a night, compared with those sleeping ten hours.[8]

• A Spanish study of 1,772 adolescents (15 years or older) reported an association between short sleep duration and obesity.[9]

• In a French study of 1,031 children aged five years, children sleeping less than 11 hours a night were significantly more obese.[10]

• A study of 11–16-year-olds in Texas determined that lack of sleep had a profound influence on daytime physical-activity levels. Daytime physical activity diminished by 3 per cent for every hour of sleep lost. Worse, for each hour of lost sleep, the odds of obesity increased by 80 per cent.[11]

Kids, TV and sleep

Regular television viewing is associated with altered sleep patterns and sleep disorders, especially amongst children and adolescents.[12] No one has the definitive answer as to how TV can interfere with sleep, but there are several theories.[13]

One is that TV may have an actual physiological impact on its viewers: the bright light of the television before sleep affects the sleep/wake cycle through suppression of the release of the hormone melatonin.[14] This effect is relevant for people of all ages. Another theory is that television may have a psychological impact on its viewers. Children in particular may watch programmes that are developmentally inappropriate for their ages or that have a violent content, and this may inhibit the relaxation necessary for sound sleep. A third potential explanation is that parents of children who watch significant amounts of television are simply poor limit-setters, unable or unwilling to enforce rules with regard to both television viewing and regular sleep times.

While TV is not the single answer to childhood obesity, limiting your child's access to it, especially at night, may have a knock-on effect on health in both the short and the long term.

Sleep regulates metabolism

The question that has vexed scientists is: how does a short sleep duration impact on body weight?

We are only just beginning to explore and understand the deep links between sleep, appetite and metabolism. What is emerging is that sleep debt interferes with the way our bodies digest and process food. There is good evidence that sleep deprivation can adversely affect glucose tolerance,[15] as well as glucose and insulin regulation.[16]

Research at the University of Chicago in 1999, published in *The Lancet*, found that after four hours of sleep for six consecutive nights, healthy young men had blood-test results that nearly matched those of diabetics.[17] Their ability both to secrete insulin and to respond to insulin decreased by about 30 per cent;

a similar decrease in immediate insulin response after a meal is an early marker of diabetes. Their bodies also took 40 per cent longer than normal to regulate their blood-sugar levels following a high-carbohydrate meal.

In the same study, sleep deprivation also altered the production and action of other key hormones in the study participants, dampening the secretion of the thyroid-stimulating hormone and increasing blood levels of the stress hormone cortisol (see pages 146–149), especially during the afternoon and evening. Elevated evening cortisol levels are typical of much older subjects, and are thought to be linked to age-related health problems, such as insulin resistance and memory impairment. All these abnormalities returned to normal during the recovery period, when subjects spent 12 hours in bed.

Given these findings, some scientists are now suggesting that an inexpensive and effective way to improve the health of people with type-2 diabetes might be simply to improve the duration and quality of their sleep.

Available research also suggests that two opposing hormones involved in the regulation of appetite, leptin and ghrelin, are disrupted by lack of sleep. Leptin (see pages 32–35) is produced by adipocytes (fat cells) to signal the state of fat stores, while ghrelin is released by the stomach to signal hunger. Low leptin and high ghrelin levels signal an energy deficit to the hypothalamus in the brain, resulting in hunger, thus motivating the body to increase food intake.

Recently researchers at the University of Bristol analysed blood samples from people suffering from insomnia and compared them with ones from those who slept well. They found that those with disrupted sleep patterns had levels of leptin that were 15 per cent lower than normal, and levels of ghrelin that were 15 per cent higher than normal. The balance between these two hormones is crucial in controlling appetite and metabolism. The researchers suggested that, especially in societies with easy access to high-calorie foods, the skewed ratio of these hormones in sleep-deprived individuals may make a substantial contribution to the development of obesity.[18]

In another more recent study, researchers followed more than 120,000 people for ten years, looking at the relationship between self-reported sleep duration and the chance of being diagnosed with diabetes over that period. Short sleepers (those who slept less than five hours per night) had a 57 per cent higher risk of developing diabetes compared to those who slept for around eight hours nightly, who had no increased risk. Interestingly, those who slept for more than nine hours each night also had an increased risk; they were 47 per cent more likely to develop diabetes during the course of the study.[19]

Even after taking into account all other factors, such as weight and age, the risk remained significant, with those sleeping less than five hours per night having a 37 per cent increased risk of diabetes, compared to those who slept eight hours per night, who had no increased risk.

The impact of snoring

An often-overlooked cause of sleep disruption and weight gain is snoring: either your own or your partner's. It is estimated that in the US 9 per cent of women and 24 per cent of men who suffer from sleep apnoea (where you stop breathing periodically in the night) also suffer from Metabolic Syndrome.[20]

Being kept awake by another person's snoring can trigger all the hormone deficits and surpluses of regular sleep deprivation and lead to the same weight-gain consequences. However, if you are the snorer, other metabolic changes may be taking place on top of these. Habitual snoring has been independently linked to obesity, poor academic performance, daytime sleepiness, hypertension, stroke and heart disease.

According to recent research at the Naval Medical Center in San Diego, which examined the records of more than 4,800 snorers, obesity and snoring were on average linked in 73 per cent of cases. What was surprising, however, was that the louder a person snores and the longer the duration of the snoring during the night, the greater the risk of obesity.[21]

Many studies into snoring and obesity confirm that disordered breathing during sleep exerts a profound effect on the body, by disrupting not only hormone levels, but also the function of the central and sympathetic nervous system.[22] It is this multisystem effect on the body that links snoring to Metabolic Syndrome. If you suffer from obstructive sleep apnoea, it can trigger the sympathetic nervous system to increase the heart rate and blood pressure. These periodic arousals of sympathetic-nervous-system activation also lead to poor insulin control.

Count sheep, not calories

While the data suggesting that lack of sleep can cause weight gain is convincing, little effort has been made by the scientific community to confirm that more and better sleep will help you lose weight. Nevertheless the idea is gaining ground.

According to Dr Kenneth Goodrick, a psychologist at Baylor College of Medicine in Houston:

Sleep is a vital component in a three-step cycle which I call 'an energy enhancement approach to weight management'. This approach looks at sleep, nutrition and exercise as the foundation for high 'perceived' energy. Overweight people often suffer from breathing problems while sleeping, which interrupts the sleep cycle. Sleep deprivation has been found to upset the glucose metabolism and sets people up for increased risk for obesity and diabetes.[23]

Goodrick has gone on record saying that sleep is the first component for his weight-management approach. He believes that lack of sleep – for instance, from snoring and night-time breathing problems – robs people of the energy they need to exercise and sets up a vicious low-energy cycle that sabotages conventional weight-loss programmes.

As energy levels drop, people turn to high-fat and high-sugar foods or caffeinated beverages for an energy pick-me-up. Some may drink 10–15 caffeinated beverages a day, and these in turn have a devastating effect on sleep quality.

Exercise, on the other hand, has an energizing effect. However, we need to have energy in order to be motivated to exercise. In treating obesity, Goodrick says, the goal is to raise energy levels through good sleep and nutrition, so that people will want to stay active. He believes his energy-enhancement approach works best when people get about eight hours of sleep.

A vicious cycle

Snoring can make obesity worse, and obesity can increase the problem of snoring.

If the snorer is overweight, losing weight may help to eliminate some of the fat in the throat, thus clearing the breathing passages. But it is worth considering what else may be causing the snoring. Allergies, for instance, cause snoring (they can also cause weight gain, see pages 125–126), so you might want to investigate whether the problem is food, dander (animal scales), chemicals or airborne allergens. Alcohol consumption close to bedtime can also exacerbate snoring.

Researchers in Canada agree. A 2005 study at Laval University in Quebec found that there may be an 'ideal sleep zone' of around eight hours a night that facilitates body-weight regulation.[24] The findings of the study, which involved 323 men and 417 women, showed that those who were 'normal sleepers' – getting between seven and eight hours of sleep per night – had lower body weight and less body fat than short sleepers who only got five to six hours of sleep a night. The analysis also demonstrated that the majority of short sleepers (88 per cent) had lower levels of circulating leptin than the normal sleepers.

The authors concluded: 'Getting the optimal amount of sleep, along with modifications to diet and exercise, may become an integral prevention and treatment strategy for weight management.'

The importance of relaxation

The healthiest people understand the value of taking a break – not just once a year, but every day and at the weekend. They generally have hobbies and interests that absorb them fully, and schedule time for these in their lives. They also take regular holidays, and value – indeed, actively pursue – time with family and friends. Such individuals do for themselves what most 'stress-management' experts make a lot of money teaching; they learn to spread the load, switch off and recharge their emotional batteries from time to time.

But you can also relax simply by having a change of scene, listening to music or going to the movies, or taking a walk in the

67

park. Equally, you can schedule relaxation time – for instance, by having regular massage or sauna sessions. Whichever way you do it, the benefits will be manifold.

Relaxation lowers levels of stress hormones and boosts immunity. It slows your heart rate and deepens your breathing.[25] Formal types of relaxation, such as Transcendental Meditation, have been shown to reduce hypertension and oxidative stress (caused by an excess of the rogue molecules known as free-radicals),[26] raise blood concentrations of the stress-busting hormone dehydroepiandrosterone sulphate (DHEAS)[27] and improve symptoms of chronic pain syndromes (which can also be associated with obesity).[28]

Insomnia

The usual symptoms of insomnia are familiar: difficulty in falling asleep, waking up frequently during the night and then finding it hard to return to sleep, or waking up 'too early' in the morning. But whilst most of us would define insomnia by the number of hours of sleep 'lost' in a night, in fact it can also defined by the quality of the sleep we normally get. If you sleep throughout the night, but still wake unrefreshed, you may be also be suffering from insomnia and it may be affecting your health in myriad ways.

Insomnia can be a signal of a body that is breaking down, and several of the health disorders that have long been blamed on obesity are also linked to insomnia. For example, chronic insomnia can herald the onset of a serious illness, such as heart disease, which is twice as prevalent in poor sleepers. Insomniacs are also three times more likely to develop frequent debilitating headaches. Other conditions that insomnia may presage include arthritis, kidney disease, heart failure, asthma, Parkinson's disease and hyperthyroidism.

Surveys show that fewer than half of insomniacs ever go to their doctor for help, and in truth consulting a doctor may be of limited value. Medical training devotes limited time and attention to the problem of insomnia, which may explain why the advice and treatment offered frequently seem so limited.

Insomnia can affect people of all ages, although it is more likely among the over-sixties, women in general and post-menopausal women in particular. There are three different grades of insomnia. Those who suffer bouts of insomnia that last from just one night to several weeks have what is called 'transient insomnia'. If your sleep patterns are disturbed only from time to time, you have 'intermittent insomnia'. However, if your insomnia occurs on most nights and lasts for a month or more, you are suffering from 'chronic insomnia'.

If your insomnia is transient or intermittent, it is unlikely your doctor will prescribe anything to help. Instead he or she may dole out the usual advice, such as taking a warm bath before bed, reading a book (provided it is boring), listening to calming music and drinking a cup of camomile tea. You may be advised not to do any exercise up to four hours before going to bed, not to eat a heavy meal just before bedtime and to avoid caffeine and alcohol in the evening.

For chronic insomnia, you may be given a tranquilliser such as benzodiazepine, or an antidepressant, if depression is the main cause of your sleeplessness. Benzodiazepines are the most commonly prescribed drugs for insomnia, but even our normally prescription-happy doctors generally do not like to prescribe a course of more than four weeks. Most know that insomnia is a symptom, rather than a disease, and pills can only work for a short time and may become addictive; ironically tranquillizers are also amongst the prescription drugs most associated with increased weight gain (see pages 106–111).

Whatever type of insomnia you have, solving it will require a commitment to investigating, in a more detailed way, exactly what in your lifestyle may be causing the problem.

How to get to sleep

Relaxation can aid a good night's sleep. But sleep and relaxation are not the same thing. Sleep is an active state that is essential for physical and mental restoration. These days, many of us simply don't get enough of it, either because we do not recognize its importance or because we have trouble falling asleep, even when we're tired (this occurs in around 30 per cent of the adult population).

Under normal circumstances we spend one-third of our lives in bed, so getting the most from your sleep time is possibly the simplest way to improve your health and your resistance to many of the toxic elements that you encounter each day. To get a better night's sleep, consider the following:

• Bedrooms are for sleeping. Remove all distractions from your bedroom, including TVs, computers, bills to be paid and any work brought home from the office.

• Keep your sleep schedule consistent. Plan regular hours of sleep each day, then stick to the programme.

• Don't exercise or involve yourself in difficult mental tasks near bedtime. However, a daily exercise regime can reduce stress, which in turn can help with insomnia.

• Don't drink before bedtime. It is a myth that alcohol helps us sleep. Instead, it temporarily depresses the nervous system and is then rapidly metabolized, causing a rebound stimulation a few hours later. Caffeine and cigarettes also keep you awake, if you have them too close to bedtime.

• Have a snack. Low blood sugar can sometimes cause you to wake in the night. Eating a high-carbohydrate food – such as a slice of bread or wholegrain crackers – or a banana before bedtime can help. A complex-carbohydrate snack can also significantly increase levels of the hormone serotonin, which helps to reduce anxiety and promote sleep.

• Open a window as fresh air can be an aid to refreshing sleep.

• Is it time to replace the mattress? Your mattress should provide firm support to your body throughout the night. Soft, sagging mattresses can lead to backache, sleeplessness and stress. Although expensive, the newer varieties of latex rubber mattresses, or those made from space-age materials such as Tempur, have many advantages over sprung types, including firmness, the ability to mould their shape to your body, lower levels of dust mites and no metal parts to attract EMFs to the bed.

• Is it an allergy? Food allergies or intolerances can cause insomnia, especially in children. Studies show about a six-hour delay between eating the offending food and a feeling of being wide awake – probably due to an outpouring of various hormones that interfere with sleep.

• Deal with stress, through counselling and other techniques, such as yoga and meditation. Many trials have shown that psychological intervention can be helpful for insomnia (see also pages 152–155).

• Quit smoking. Studies show that smokers are more likely to suffer from insomnia than non-smokers.

• Supplement your diet. Because stress takes its toll on the body's nutritional supplies, try taking calcium (100 mg daily) together with magnesium (200–500 mg daily): the combination may produce a tranquillizing effect. Stress can deplete levels of B vitamins, so supplement with a B-complex that includes 50–100 mg of the entire family of B nutrients.

• Try herbal remedies, which certainly come with fewer adverse effects than prescription drugs. These include valerian, passiflora, St John's wort, camomile, hops and catnip. Likewise, research suggests that sprinkling lavender oil on your pillow works just as well as tranquillizers.

• Cut the caffeine. The effects of caffeine can last for up to 20 hours, so some people will have disturbed sleep patterns even when their last cup of coffee was in the morning. Watch for hidden caffeine in tea, green tea, soft drinks, chocolate and over-the-counter drugs.

Embracing the darkness

One way in which you can increase your melatonin production is to make certain that you sleep in an absolutely dark environment. The normal daily rhythm of intense sunlight alternating with nights of near-total darkness has dominated life on Earth for many thousands of years. We have altered this cycle recently with artificial lights that can bombard city dwellers around the clock. This can lead to melatonin disturbances that can affect how well we sleep, and which may also raise the risk of developing cancer.

Early evidence linking light to cancer emerged in the 1990s from studies into blind women who are not sensitive to changes in light, and whose melatonin levels consequently do not change. These studies showed an approximately 20–50 per cent reduced risk of breast cancer among such women[29] over normally sighted women. The more profoundly blind the women, the lower their risk of developing cancer.[30]

Heavy curtains or blinds should be a priority in bedrooms or, if this is not possible, try using eye masks to keep your eyes from registering light when they should be registering darkness. Getting rid of night-lights is also a good idea. If you need to get up in the night, try not to turn on lights, as this will disrupt normal melatonin production.

In modern society where sleep can be in short supply, improving your sleep habits and the quality of your sleep can represent a substantial step forward in managing your weight. Healing a body overwhelmed by exhaustion is something that most of us can do without the help of a professional. Not so the problem of a body overwhelmed by pollution, as the next chapter reveals.

CHAPTER 4

The problem of 'chemical calories'

Your body is constantly being exposed to a range of substances that can accumulate, particularly in fat cells, and lead to a state of chronic toxicity. Some of these, such as the pollutants we breathe and the herbicides and pesticides that lace many of the foods we eat, come from the outside. Many of them are present in and on products that we use every day. Others are the result of the metabolic and physiological processes that go on in our bodies each day.

The body does not like to let the concentration of potentially harmful substances rise too high. As a result, it has evolved numerous ways to process and eliminate from its system unwanted, naturally occurring substances – for instance, through sweat and urine. But the body can easily become overwhelmed by man-made toxins that it was never meant to deal with; and when it can't metabolize certain man-made toxins quickly enough, it tries to deal with them in other ways.

One way is to dilute them by hanging on to excess fluid. Fluid retention (which can produce swollen ankles, puffy hands and face) is a common factor in food intolerance, which is itself a frequent underlying feature of chronic toxicity. It is also common in chemical poisoning.

The other way in which the body deals with toxic chemicals is by diluting them in fat. Many man-made chemicals have an affinity with fat; they are naturally attracted to the fat that is contained within the fat cells around the body. And, purely from the perspective of survival, this storage capacity makes perfect sense, since it keeps the circulating levels of otherwise-toxic substances out of the system and away from vital organs like the heart, lungs, kidneys and liver.

Storing toxins in these ways can obviously encourage weight gain. But toxins can also make us fat in other ways. For instance, some may interfere with the body's metabolic reactions, causing them to stall and thus encouraging weight to accumulate. Given this, many people would say that losing weight as quickly as possible would be the healthiest way to get rid of accumulated toxins, and therefore of fat. However, once your body becomes overwhelmed with man-made chemicals, it just isn't that simple.

As already outlined in this book, fast weight loss and ongoing fluctuations in weight are hard on the body. People who do not maintain a stable weight throughout life are at greater risk of dying prematurely from a range of diseases.

With regard to the accumulation of harmful chemicals in the body, scientists are now speculating that there is yet another reason why repeated fluctuations in weight may do more harm than good. As we lose body fat, stored toxins are released into the bloodstream. The amounts released can become quite significant with the repeated weight losses of yo-yo dieting.

This fact was brought home in the late 1990s in data

presented by Dr Roy Walford, a researcher on ageing at the University of California in Los Angeles, at a meeting of the American Association for the Advancement of Science.

In 1999 Walford tested blood samples that he collected from scientists who participated in a two-year experiment known as Biosphere 2 – a prototype self-sustaining, greenhouse-like capsule in the Arizona desert.[1] He measured blood levels of PCBs (polychlorinated biphenyls: industrial coolants and conductors, now banned because of their toxicity) and DDE (a breakdown product of the pesticide DDT) in the blood of the four men and four women participating in the project, including himself. These persistent synthetic chemicals, once widely used in industry and agriculture, are known to exert adverse effects on the nervous system, and have also been linked to cancer.

During the two years that the participants lived in the Biosphere they ate a predominantly vegetarian, nutrient-dense diet of fruits and vegetables grown inside the capsule. They also ate small amounts of goat meat and milk, pork, chicken, fish and eggs. Due to unexpected food shortages, they lost significant amounts of weight, particularly during the first six to nine months of the project. On average, the men lost 18 per cent of their body weight, while the women lost 10 per cent.

Analysis of their blood samples taken during the period of most dramatic weight loss revealed that blood levels of toxins increased as much as fivefold. The toxins gradually cleared from the bloodstream as their weight stabilized during the second year. However, as Walford pointed out, losing weight again and again could repeat the process over and over, releasing significant amounts of toxins into the bloodstream. Once there, these substances are free to attack vulnerable organs and body tissues – just another reason, it would seem, to lose weight slowly, and keep it off.

Hormone havoc

There are many ways in which man-made chemicals can interfere with weight control. Amongst the most devastating are those that interfere with the body's naturally occurring hormones.

The endocrine or hormonal system is composed of many different organs and glands – such as the pituitary, hypothalamus, thyroid and adrenal glands, the pancreas, thymus, ovaries and testes – that produce and secrete a variety of unique hormones directly into the bloodstream.

Once in the bloodstream, hormones travel to special 'receptors' throughout the body. Each type of hormone has a specific target, or receptor, that it must connect with in order to transmit its information. Hormones are essentially chemical messengers transmitting information between cells. The interaction between hormone and receptor is vital to maintaining optimal hormone levels, as well as controlling normal physiological processes and maintaining the body's natural state of balance. However, this balance can be thrown out by the presence of chemical interlopers – synthetic hormones, or hormone mimics, that can interfere with the normal interplay between hormones and can target organs and receptor cells within the body.

Once in the body, these hormonally active agents can mimic or interfere with the actions of almost any hormone-producing gland. Because of this, exposure to industrial chemicals – many of which are known hormone mimics – may have a role to play in a range of common disorders, such as hypothyroidism (underactivity of the thyroid gland), diabetes mellitus and hypoglycaemia (low blood-glucose levels), as well as reproductive disorders and cancer.

Hormones also play a major role in determining and maintaining metabolism and the body's set point (see page 20).

When levels of these hormones (produced by the thyroid, the sympathetic nervous system and the reproductive organs) deviate from the norm, problems with weight can ensue.

Thus, in January 2004, at a conference entitled 'Obesity: Developmental Origins and Environmental Influences', the US National Institutes of Health made a demand for more research into the link between hormone-disrupting chemicals and obesity, noting that exposure during adulthood and, crucially, in the womb can permanently disrupt the body's weight-control mechanisms.[2]

Up until that point, many scientists believed that the influence of industrial chemicals (and in particular hormone-disrupting substances) on weight management was unproven. However, according to at least one scientist, the research has been there for years, albeit hidden between the lines of the data. In 2002 Dr Paula Baillie-Hamilton, a visiting Fellow at the Occupational and Environmental Health Research Group, Stirling University, Scotland, published a paper in which she proposed that chemical toxins were to blame for the global obesity epidemic.[3]

Baillie-Hamilton's hypothesis, the culmination of many years of forensic investigation into the way that pollution is changing us from the inside out, had its roots in an article that she stumbled upon, which explained how toxic chemicals in the environment were affecting the fertility of wildlife. 'I couldn't understand how someone like myself, an academic with a load of different scientific qualifications and papers behind me, had never heard of all these different chemicals that were out there,' she commented in a recent interview:

Yet if these chemicals were affecting the fertility of wildlife, they must be affecting hormones to a significant degree. And of course hormones control a number of other functions in the body, including weight control.

There were no books available on the subject, so I spent a couple of years intensively identifying each major category of chemical and working out how each individual substance affected the body's weight-control system. I looked at all the mechanisms involved, from the nerves and hormones to metabolism and the levels of nutrients in the body, and found that the same chemicals that at high doses can cause weight loss, seemed to cause a fattening effect at very low levels – the same low levels that we are exposed to in everyday life.[4]

It was an arduous task made more difficult by the fact that weight gain is not always documented in trials of toxic chemicals. For many years this data has been ignored or suppressed in the conclusions of scientific papers, because there was no way to explain why it happened, and of course it was not accepted at the time that weight gain in animals exposed to toxic substances like DDT could be anything other than positive. Indeed, if weight gain was mentioned, it would be buried in the text of the paper, rather than the conclusion, which means that unless you were looking specifically for this effect, you would never really find it.

A chemical cosh

Industrial chemicals – and specifically those that act like hormone-disrupters – profoundly alter several aspects of human metabolism and appetite control.

Research at the University of Laval in Quebec has added greatly to our understanding of just how wide-ranging the effects of a polluted body can be. In the late 1990s – around the time that the Biosphere tests were published – Professor Angelo Tremblay and his team began to study, first in animals and then in people, the metabolic effects of organochlorines – for instance, the pesticides DDT (and its breakdown product DDE), chlordane, aldrin, dieldrin and heptachlor and the now-banned industrial lubricants PCBs, as well as dioxins and chlorophenols.

Their interest was sparked by earlier Italian research,[5] which showed that overweight people who underwent gastric bypasses to encourage weight loss experienced dramatic increases in levels of the pesticide DDT and one of its breakdown products, DDE, in their blood as their body weight declined. The Laval studies of humans undergoing an average weight-loss programme also showed that concentrations of these chemicals rose as the pounds were shed.[6]

Once in the body, organochlorines and other industrial pollutants are generally stored in human fat cells. During weight loss the fat cells shrink and release these chemicals back into the bloodstream. The scientists at Laval found that as levels of these now freely circulating pollutants rose in dieters, so the levels of essential thyroid hormones – necessary for maintaining an efficient metabolism – fell dramatically.

A drop in basal metabolic rate (the rate at which the body burns calories) is not uncommon in dieters. Studies into weight loss show that as metabolism slows down during weight loss, levels of thyroid hormones also drop naturally. This slowdown is referred to as 'adaptive thermogenesis'.

The worrying discovery of the Laval scientists was that higher levels of organochlorine compounds were associated with much lower levels of thyroid hormones than would be produced by weight loss alone. In dieters with these newly liberated toxins circulating throughout the body, the basal metabolic rate also slowed dramatically, as did energy expenditure and levels of skeletal muscle oxidative enzymes (which determine how efficiently the muscles use energy – when levels are below optimum, energy gets stored as fat).

To put this in lay terms, organochlorines essentially shut down the metabolic furnace that helps the body burn fat.

The Canadian research has focused on organochlorine compounds, but the list of chemicals that can cause weight gain and promote obesity extends well beyond these, to include a wide variety of everyday chemicals associated with manufacturing and a dirty environment (see box on pages 84–86).

A key effect is the way that industrial pollutants interact with the sympathetic nervous system. This system releases hormones like adrenaline and noradrenaline that suppress our appetite, particularly for fat. These hormones also increase the ability and desire to exercise, as well as increasing body temperature, so that while you are exercising you are burning calories more efficiently.

Chemicals like organochlorines act directly on the sympathetic nervous system, attacking each and every part of the way it works. It is, in Paula Baillie-Hamilton's words, 'a chemical cosh' that reduces levels of the important hormones necessary for weight balance and also blocks and even destroys the hormone receptors in fat cells. This means that the hormones cannot communicate with the fat cells, and the cells becomes less sensitive to those metabolism-regulating hormones that are in circulation.

Adapt and survive

Ongoing research continues to confirm that high circulating levels of organochlorines alter metabolism and may be one of the most important contributors to adaptive thermogenesis and the rebound weight gain that is so familiar to dieters.[7]

But, once liberated by weight loss, these chemicals are also free to attack vital organs, such as the brain, liver and kidneys, and this threat triggers an even more intriguing response. As chemicals build up beyond a level with which the body's detoxification pathways can cope, the body begins to 'dilute' the amount of circulating toxins – the majority of which are fat-soluble – by making new fat cells to store them in.

Recent research even shows that the presence of some industrial pollutants such as bisphenol-A and organotins can signal dormant 'baby' fat cells, known as preadipocytes, to grow into fully mature fat cells, or adipocytes.[8] As the number of fat cells increases, it can become harder to keep weight down. In addition, with increasing weight, the body detoxification system, which would normally facilitate the excretion of toxins, appears to shut down, in preference to simply storing any toxins in available fat.[9]

There is still much that is unknown about the way these chemicals interfere with metabolism, but apart from triggering hormonal changes, the presence of organochlorines and other toxins can also act as allergens and inflammatory triggers (see also pages 129–132).

Although we think of fat as pathogenic, or capable of causing disease, the way in which the body responds to chronic toxicity by diluting the chemicals in fat is really a protective effect. For example, studies show that animals that are exposed to environmental toxins while simultaneously being encouraged to gain weight through a high-calorie diet will survive better than exposed animals that are not allowed to gain weight. In other words, body fat – because it is a repository of these toxins – also becomes a survival mechanism. Thus it is possible that the obesity 'epidemic' is really an adaptive response by the body to a chemically toxic environment.

Viewed in this way, obesity could be seen as the response of an intelligent body trying to cope and maintain balance in an overwhelmingly polluted world. Sadly, in an environment where we are overwhelmed with pollutants, this intelligent adaptation brings its own threat to continued good health; and continued advice to simply decrease one's calorie intake dramatically in order to speed weight loss may even be making the problem worse.[10]

Chemical calories

In addition to organochlorines, a range of other industrial and everyday chemicals is known to encourage weight gain. These include:

Organophosphates[11]
Organophosphate pesticides, such as malathion, dursban, diazinon and carbonates, constitute 40 per cent of all pesticides used. These chemicals are mainly utilized inside buildings, as opposed to in agriculture. They are neurotoxic (harmful to nerve tissue) and hormone-disrupting.

Carbamates[12]
Including aldicarb, bendiocarb, carbaryl, propoxur and thiophanate methyl, carbamates are used extensively in agriculture, forestry and gardening. They are suspected hormone-disrupters.

Organotins[13]
These include tributyltin (TBT) and the mono- and dibutyltins (MBT, DBT). These chemicals have many applications, including as stabilizers in PVC, catalysts in chemical reactions. They are also found in glass coatings, agricultural pesticides, biocides in marine

anti-foulant paints and wood treatments and preservatives.
Organotins are damaging to the thyroid and immune system and
potential hormone-disrupters.

Bisphenol-A[14]

An oestrogen mimic used to make clear, hard, reusable plastic
products; it is also used in the manufacture of polymers, fungicides,
antioxidants, dyes, polyester resins, flame-retardants and rubber
chemicals, and some dental resins.

Phthalates[15]

Hormone-disrupting chemicals, these are produced in large volumes
and are commonly detected in ground water, rivers and drinking
water, as well as in meat and dairy products. Around 95 per cent of
phthalate production over the last few decades has been tied to the
PVC industry. Phthalates can be found in many plastics and
consumer products – everything from hair spray and nail varnish to
plastic water bottles and T-shirts.

Polybrominated flame-retardants[16]

These are added to many products, including computers, TVs and
household textiles to reduce fire risk. They are also found in baby
mattresses, foam mattresses, car seats and PVC products. Office
workers who use computers, hospital cleaners and workers in
electronics-dismantling plants are at particular risk from these
chemicals. Polybrominated flame-retardants are oestrogen mimics
and can also affect the thyroid.

Benzo[a]pyrene[17]

A common food pollutant that belongs to a family of chemicals
known as polycyclic aromatic hydrocarbons (PAHs). It is derived from
coal tar and enters the atmosphere as a result of incomplete

combustion of fossil fuels. In animals it has been shown to cause weight gain in the absence of any detectable change in food intake. It is possible that other PAHs may have a similar effect.

Solvents[18]

Neurotoxic chemicals that include xylene, dichlorobenzene, ethylphenol, styrene, toluene, acetone and trichloroethane are commonly found in human blood samples. They are necessary for a wide range of industrial processes and are found widely in adhesives, glues, cleaning fluids, felt-tip pens, perfumes, paints, varnishes, pesticides, petrol, household cleaners and waxes.

Cadmium[19]

This is principally used as a protective plating for steel, in electrode material in nickel-cadmium batteries and as a component of various alloys. It is also present in phosphate fertilizers, fungicides and pesticides. Cadmium in the soil is taken up through the roots of plants and distributed to edible leaves, fruits and seeds, and is eventually passed on to humans and other animals, where it can build up in milk and fatty tissues. Cadmium is neurotoxic and a potential hormone-disrupter.

Lead[20]

Professions that put their employees at risk of exposure to this neurotoxin include lead-smelting, -refining and -manufacturing industries, brass/bronze foundries, the rubber and plastics industries, steel-welding and -cutting operations, and battery manufacturing plants. Construction workers and people who work in municipal waste incinerators, in the pottery and ceramics industries, radiator-repair shops and other industries that use lead solder may also be among high-exposure groups.

Uncomfortable questions

Overweight and obesity represent a global problem and are definitely associated with industrialization and pollution. In September 2006 a 'fat map' of Britain was published by Dr Foster Intelligence, an independent health-research organization that works closely with the National Health Service and with Experian, a market-research company.

The analysis was a complex synthesis of data from two surveys – the Health Survey for England, and the British Market Research Bureau's quarterly survey of 25,000 Britons – which provided details of lifestyle and Body Mass Index (BMI, the indication of how overweight a person is; but see pages 26–27) and geographical location. Its conclusion was that people living in northern industrial towns were fatter than those living in London and in other, more rural areas of the UK.[21] The most overweight people in this survey were living largely in the industrial north of the UK, where once there were mines, refineries, factories and tall chimneys belching out smoke, and where now there are chemical factories, incinerators and waste-transfer facilities regularly releasing toxins into the air, water and soil.

This scenario is not unique to Britain. A 2006 survey by the Trust for America's Health found that the ten fattest states in the US – Mississippi, Alabama, West Virginia, Louisiana, Kentucky, Tennessee, Arkansas, Indiana, South Carolina and Texas, were located in the industrial south of the nation.[22] The report failed to mention any aspect of the environment, yet the Mississippi River, which runs through several of these states, is officially the most polluted river in the US.[23] Likewise, West Virginia, Texas, Indiana, Alabama, Louisiana and Georgia are home to some of the top 20 mercury-polluting power plants.[24] Fish and wildlife in some southern states like Alabama, Arkansas and Tennessee are regularly found to be contaminated by organochlorines like DDT and PCBs – due to the former production of these chemicals in these areas.

Of course there may be confounding factors, because industrialization and pollution are also associated with dietary changes and alterations in activity patterns. Nevertheless, clinical practice has been frustratingly slow to catch up with the conceptual changes demanded by the link between environmental pollutants and obesity.

The health problems associated with polluted bodies are usually unseen. Some, like cancer or Alzheimer's disease, can take decades to develop. The problems of overweight and obesity offer us a rare and very visible clue that tells us that pollution may be killing us, inch by ever-expanding inch.

Nevertheless, if you are talking to an obesity specialist – whose entire life's work has been spent telling people that if they eat too much and don't exercise they are going to gain weight – you may not get much insight into the link between industrial pollutants and weight gain. Yet until our doctors do begin to understand more about the influence of chemical toxins, their conclusions (and the solutions they propose) will continue to be very limited.

The recognition that chemical pollutants could have such a direct effect on our bodies is possibly one of the most important new ideas in public health, and one that demands a difficult, but necessary shift in our conceptual understanding of the dynamics of weight control. Allied to this there is an urgent need to acknowledge the way that our actions shape our environment, and in which our environment, in turn, shapes our lives.

Children at risk

Children are many times more vulnerable to the effects of toxic insults than adults, in part because their response to toxic exposure is often very different from that of adults. Good examples of this are the paradoxical responses to phenobarbital and methylphenidate (Ritalin) in children compared with adults. Phenobarbital acts like a sedative in adults, but produces hyperactivity in children; Ritalin, a cocaine-like drug, is used as an anti-hyperactivity drug in children, but has a stimulant effect in adults.

There are many reasons for this paradoxical response. But perhaps the most influential is that infants and children are still growing and developing. During childhood, different systems and organs develop at different rates and in different phases. Growing tissue may be much more sensitive to toxic exposure than other tissue. Indeed, studies of exposure to cigarette smoke have shown that the risk of dying of breast cancer is greater for those who started smoking before the age of 16 than for those who started smoking after the age of 20.[25]

In addition to growing and developing, children differ from adults in a number of other ways that can increase their susceptibility to toxins.[26] For example:
• Their body systems have a less-developed ability to break down toxins[27]
• They eat, drink and breathe more for their weight than adults, which means that they take in more toxins per kg (2.2 lb) than adults – for example, the air intake of a resting infant is twice that of an adult under the same conditions
• They crawl around on the floor near dust and other potentially toxic particles

• They are more likely to put things in their mouths and eat things that they shouldn't.

Children's bodies may also have less capacity to repair damage. In addition, the developing foetus is extremely sensitive to the complex interactions of signalling chemicals (hormones). Disruption of these hormonal signals can permanently skew the body's development on many fronts, including the proper development of its weight-management systems.

Keeping chemicals at bay

For many years chronic exposure to low levels of poisons in the environment was associated primarily with allergies or 'intolerance' in humans – a catch-all term often used to describe a collection of seemingly unrelated symptoms. As research in this area progressed, it became clear that with the rising level of environmental assaults on the body, the impact of environmental toxins was much broader than that, producing a wide range of symptoms that extend beyond the allergy model. New medical diagnoses such as 'sick building syndrome'[28] and 'multiple chemical sensitivity'[29] began to emerge.

The chemicals involved in these disorders were found to be neurotoxic and disruptive to the endocrine and immune systems, and it took only a small leap of logic for physicians to begin to speculate that, left unattended, these initial vague symptoms could, over time, develop into more serious diseases later in life, such as heart disease, autoimmune disorders and even cancer.

We now know more than ever before about the things in our environment that have the potential to make us ill.[30, 31] Typically these include:

• Airborne pollutants, such as benzenes, xylenes and other

solvents and volatile organic compounds (VOCs) – common in perfumes, petrol and other consumer products, as well as in industrial fall-out

• Endocrine-disrupters, present in pesticides, plastics, toiletries, flame-retardants and industrial pollution, such as dioxins and PCBs

• Pesticides found in and on foods, but also in our water supply (for instance, fluoride began life as a pesticide) and in the air

• Heavy metals, such as dental fillings containing mercury, as well as fish and food preservatives and cosmetics.

So compelling is the evidence that a specialist field – environmental medicine or, more formally clinical ecology – has evolved to assess the impact of these environmental factors on health, and to treat those suffering from what is broadly termed 'environmental illness'.

The field of environmental medicine is largely acknowledged to have begun with the clinical observations of Dr Theron Randolph in the 1960s. Randolph is known as the founding father of environmental medicine, and many of his works remain standard references even today.[32] However, it is really in the last decade that the field has burgeoned and penetrated a wider consciousness. Today it is a speciality practised by more than 3,000 physicians worldwide, most of them in the US and Britain, as well as Canada and Australia.

While we all carry these toxins in our bodies to a greater or lesser extent, some groups such as children, women (especially pregnant women) and the elderly are more affected than others.[33] It seems incredible that we could be exposed to so many pollutants on a regular basis, but you don't have to do anything more energetic than simply move through your day in order to be exposed to a multitude of environmental toxins.

Below is a list of ways in which we all encounter a wide range of toxins, including hormone-disrupting chemicals, on a daily basis. Women taking the contraceptive pill or hormone replacement therapy (HRT) (see Chapter 5 for more on prescription drugs and weight gain) should be aware that they are already significantly hormone-disrupted even *before* they encounter these other synthetic oestrogens and hormone mimics.

1 Tap water

The endocrine-disrupting chemicals most commonly found in water include: alkylphenols and alkylphenol ethoxylates; bisphenol-A; cadmium; dioxins; pharmaceutical hormones (the contraceptive pill, HRT) and their metabolites (breakdown products); lead; organochlorine pesticides (such as endosulfan, lindane, methoxychlor, atrazine, DDT); phthalates and polychlorinated biphenyls (PCBs). You drink and cook with this water, but you also wash yourself with it, and many industrial contaminants, including oestrogen mimics, can easily pass through the skin into the body during showers, baths and dishwashing.

2 Bottled water

Worries about harmful chemicals in tap water have led many people to use bottled water instead. But the plastic bottles used for bottled water may leach the endocrine-disrupter bisphenol-A into your water.[34] Similarly, there is concern that milk and juice cartons may also leach this chemical into their contents.

3 Canned food

Metal cans are lined with a plastic to prevent metal contamination. Ironically, this coating contains bisphenol-A, a powerful endocrine-disrupter that can easily leach into food.[35] Fatty foods (such as canned meats and fish in oil) may contain the highest concentrations, though studies have shown that bisphenol-A can migrate into tinned fruits and vegetables as well.[36]

4 Soya-based infant formula

Soya contains plant-based hormone mimics known as phyto-oestrogens. Infants fed exclusively soya formula consume more of these oestrogen mimics than any other group. In a typical day, such an infant will receive 11 mg of phyto-oestrogens per kg (2.2 lb) of body weight, compared with just 1 mg/kg in the average-sized adult.[37] At best, research into the potential harmful effects is sketchy and, for the moment, has only revealed subtle changes in menstrual patterns in offspring.[38] This may change over the next few years. Soya-based infant formulas may also contain high levels of thyroid-disrupting cadmium.[39] Heating formula in plastic bottles may release bisphenol-A and phthalates into the liquid. This risk is higher with older bottles that have been repeatedly scrubbed clean and sterilized.[40]

5 'Natural' plant-oestrogen supplements

We take far too many of these, both as supplements and as New Age nutriceuticals (foods that claim to, or have been engineered to, have a specific pharmaceutical effect on the body, such as lowering cholesterol), to make up for basic deficiencies in our own diets – particularly of fresh fruit and vegetables.

6 Car exhausts

Emissions from car engines contain several unhealthy chemicals. In terms of endocrine disruption, polycyclic aromatic hydrocarbons (PAHs), in particular benzo[a]pyrene, in car exhausts may be the most significant.[41] PAHs are also generated by burning incense and candles. Burning petrol may release cadmium into the atmosphere.

7 Cigarettes

Cigarette smoke is a source of hormone-disrupting cadmium and PAHs. There is also extensive documentation of the presence of multiple pesticides in tobacco products, some of which have confirmed or suspected endocrine-disrupting effects.

8 Paper products

Including paper towels, coffee filters and tampons, most paper products that are chlorine-bleached can contain dioxins. Tampons are of particular concern because they are worn inside the body. While the levels of dioxins in tampons are probably low, they can accumulate, helped by the way that women are encouraged to use tampons – for hours, sometimes whole days at a time, for several days each month, over the course of approximately half a woman's lifetime.

9 Toiletries and cosmetics

Including body lotions, hair-styling products, make-up and sunscreens, these products contain oestrogenic preservatives known as parabens[42] (ethyl-, methyl-, butyl- and propyl-parabens). Hairsprays and nail varnishes can contain phthalates. Many sunscreening agents (such as benzophenone-3, homosalate, 4-methylbenzylidene camphor (4-MBC), octyl methoxycinnamate and octyl dimethyl-PABA) are oestrogenic[43] and even more so when combined in one product.

10 Disposable nappies

The bleach used on both outer and inner materials can produce detectable levels of carcinogenic (cancer-causing) and endocrine-disrupting dioxins. The gel used in the 'super-absorbent' core of disposable nappies has been associated with a number of risks to health, including hormone disruption. It has also been linked to lower sperm counts. Recent studies have detected another endocrine-disrupting compound, tributyltin (TBT), an industrial-strength antifungal, in disposable nappies.

11 Flea collars
Of particular concern are the oestrogen-disrupting organophosphates such as diazinon, and carbamates such as carbaryl used in these products. Many flea collars are also made of PVC, another endocrine-disrupter, creating an oestrogen-disrupting double whammy for pets and those who love them.

12 Air fresheners
These completely unnecessary products (and related products, such as perfumes) contain a variety of endocrine-disrupters. For example, the fragrance ingredient musk ambrette has been found to cause atrophy of the testicles in animal studies.[44] Citral, a common substance used in both fragrances and flavours, causes enlargement of the prostate gland and is oestrogenic.[45] This has been put forward as one reason why men working in perfume- and soap-manufacturing have an increased risk of developing prostate cancer.[46] Phthalates are also common in scented products, where they are used as solvents.[47] In an analysis of the popular perfume Calvin Klein's 'Eternity', diethyl phthalate (DEP) made up more than 10 per cent of the fragrance portion of the product.[48]

13 Animal fat
Most of the endocrine-disrupting pesticides used on farms make their way into our livestock. These substances prefer to be surrounded by fat and so are stored in the animal's fat. When we eat animal fats, we ingest these harmful substances as well.

14 Non-organic foods

Similarly, when we eat conventionally produced foods such as vegetables and grains, we are ingesting the whole range of pesticides currently used on our foods during their growth and storage. These substances cannot be effectively washed off; traces will always remain.

15 Sitting at home watching TV

Wall coverings, carpets, furnishings and TVs are treated with hormone-disrupting brominated flame-retardants. In the home environment, these chemicals can rub off onto your hands and face, or off-gas into the atmosphere. Many flame-retardant chemicals are hormone-disrupters. In particular, polybrominated diphenyl ethers (PBDEs), pentabromophenol (PBP) and tetrabromobisphenol-A (TBBPA) are known to interfere with thyroid function.[49]

Certainly most of us believe we are safe from industrial chemicals, especially those that cause hormone disruption. After all, how could an average person living an average life be exposed to relevant levels of such damaging substances? Yet, as the above list shows, we live in a world awash with synthetic hormones. We eat them, drink them, breathe them and absorb them through our skin. We use them at work, at home and in the garden. They are present in soil, water, air and food.

What this means is that along with changes in the way we eat, it is worth considering changes in the way we live. In order not to invite chemicals into your life, these changes must necessarily encompass reducing your reliance on too many toxic household cleaners and toiletries, on tobacco, plastics and synthetic fibres, on convenience foods, on gardening and pet products that contain harmful pesticides, and shifting into a simpler and less toxic way of living in the world (see Chapters 8 and 9).

Detox and fasting

At the same time that you are restricting the quantity of toxins you ingest, you can also be helping your body to eliminate stored toxins.

Detoxification is an ongoing process that removes wastes and toxins from the body whether you are eating or not. In a healthy person, it is the job of the liver and kidneys to detoxify the body. Supported by a healthy lifestyle, these organs are supremely capable of doing their job.

Nevertheless, detox is a major buzzword in the health industry. Go into any health-food shop and you will find any number of 'detox in a box' products. Most of these are as useless as they are expensive.

If you wish to detox, here are some points to consider that will help you achieve a better result:

• Why do you want to detox? Have you been exposed to a specific identifiable toxin, such as dental amalgam? Do you work in a job that regularly exposes you to solvents and other VOCs? If so, over-the-counter products are unlikely to help. You should be detoxing under the supervision of a practitioner who can tailor a regime to suit your individual needs.

• There's more to detox than loose bowels and an overstimulated bladder. Most commercial detox mixtures are little more than combinations of laxative and diuretic herbs. While this may aid elimination up to a point, it does little to deal with the deeper problems of accumulated toxins – for instance, those stored in fatty tissues. What is more, long-term use of laxatives and diuretics can substantially skew the normal mineral balance of the body.

• Think green. Green foods, rather than fruit-based products, have a better reputation for aiding detox (see pages 195–196 for more information).

• Have a regular sauna. Dry or steam saunas heat the body tissues several inches below the skin, enhancing all your metabolic processes. When all of your skin's sweat glands are working well, they can perform as much detoxification as one kidney (or both). Increased sweating increases the elimination of salt and water through the skin, as the well elimination as of metals (such as nickel, copper, zinc and lead), toxic volatile hydrocarbons (including benzene, styrene, toluene, trichloroethylene and PCBs),[50] pesticides (such as DDT and DDE) and other toxins.[51]

• Keep it simple. Vast mixtures of herbs in detox formulas may not be any more effective than a carefully chosen mixture of three or four. If in doubt, always consult a qualified herbalist.

Many people combine fasts with detox regimes. Often, detox is not used just to kick-start a diet, but (in conjunction with fasting) is used in clinical practice to treat a range of disorders, such as rheumatoid arthritis,[52] high cholesterol[53] and pancreatitis.[54] Detox may also be helpful for some psychiatric disorders, such as depression and schizophrenia.[55]

In cases of extreme poisoning, such as acute exposure to PCBs, fasting may aid the process of detoxification.[56] However, there is little to suggest that, in a healthy person, fasting is necessary to boost the power of a detox.

Nevertheless, if you choose to fast, it is helpful to know that the success of a fast depends on many factors, including its type and length and your overall level of health. Contrary to popular belief, fasting is not a good way to lose weight or a permanent way to detoxify the body. It is a short-term intervention that must be followed up by good health practices in order to maintain any benefits.

At best, fasting can provide your body with a physiological break that enables it to divert more energy to the process of removing waste and restoring balance. Under proper supervision, fasting can be constructive and uplifting. Gone into without forethought and for prolonged periods of time, it can weaken and even kill.

Safe fasting

Most people can safely fast for a short period of time without doing undue harm to the body. If you are considering a short fast of three to five days, there are guidelines that can help it be more beneficial.

• Prepare for your fast the day before by making your last meal one of fruit and vegetables; some authorities recommend that your diet the day before a fast should be vegan.

• Only water should be consumed while fasting, and the quantity of water should be dictated by your thirst. You should not consume coffee, tea, juice, soft drinks, cigarettes or anything else by mouth. Herbal teas can be supportive of a fast, but they should not be sweetened.

• Fasting should not be combined with vigorous exercise, though short walks in the fresh air may be beneficial. Conserve your energy to maximize healing. Try to take a nap or two during the day.

• Avoid exposure to chemicals such as those contained in toiletries, because these add to your body's toxic burden. Instead, consider washing simply with luke-warm water.

• Try to avoid extremes of temperature. Your body temperature may drop during a fast, so make sure that you stay warm.

• If the sun is out, try to get 10–20 minutes a day of exposure.

When you are ready to break your fast, do so slowly by choosing small quantities of food (fruit and vegetables are ideal) at room temperature. Eat slowly and chew thoroughly.

When not to fast

Most authorities agree that a detox regime with or without fasting is unlikely to harm the body and can even be healthful. However, there are some situations and some people for whom fasting is not recommended. Don't detox or fast when you are stressed or depressed. Similarly, detox of a seriously polluted body can have implications for the health of vital organs, such as the kidneys and liver, so find a qualified practitioner before starting.

If you have diabetes, ulcers or liver, kidney, heart or lung disease, advanced cancer or a compromised immune system, you should not fast or take herbal remedies unless advised to do so by a qualified practitioner. Those taking medication should also not fast, as it can alter the potency of some drugs. Fasting and detox are not recommended for pregnant and breastfeeding women[57] or for infants and children.[58]

It would be easy to assume that the chemical pollution that interferes with the body's natural weight-management system is always the fault of someone or something else. But, as the next chapter shows, in a culture of magic-bullet solutions to ill health, sometimes we bring it on ourselves.

CHAPTER 5

Pills that make you plump

We live in a pill-popping culture. No matter what ails you, no matter how trivial and self-limiting and non-life-threatening your condition, there's a pill to make it 'right'.

The prevailing myth of the pill-popping culture is that without these magic bullets we'd be sad, fat, spotty, sniffly, headachy and maybe even pregnant. And even those who shun conventional medications often end up taking pills in the form of 'safe' over-the-counter medications, as well as a battery of vitamins, minerals and herbal supplements designed to produce the same effect as prescription drugs, but 'naturally'. In short, not to be taking any kind of pill is pretty unusual these days.

All drugs cause adverse effects – even the ones you can 'safely' buy over the counter – and most of us accept the trade-off of an occasional upset tummy, skin rash or headache if it means that some bigger or more immediate health problem gets 'fixed'. The problem is that the magic bullets on which we have become so universally reliant may also be shooting our normal weight-control systems to bits.

In the summer of 2007 a headline in the British newspaper *The Independent* warned: 'Huge weight gains reported by patients on prescription drugs'.[1] The story cautioned that thousands of people who take prescription medicines to treat chronic conditions such as heart disease, depression, diabetes and epilepsy were gaining large amounts of weight as an unexpected side-effect. With many of the drugs, weight gain was significant and rapid, according to the researchers.

Such was the scale of the problem that scientists at Glasgow University and the Glasgow Royal Infirmary believed that prescription drugs might even be contributing to the nation's rocketing obesity epidemic. In the Scottish study[2] olanzapine and clozapine, drugs used for psychiatric conditions, resulted in the most dramatic weight gain: up to 10 kg (22 lb) in a year. Insulin for type-2 diabetes was found to increase weight by up to 6 kg (13¼ lb), while some drugs for depression added up to 3.6 kg (8 lb), and some for high blood pressure led to gains of up to 1.3 kg (3 lb). A heart drug added 2 kg (4½ lb), while some treatments for epilepsy added more than 5.5 kg (12 lb), and some bipolar drugs led to weight gains of around 3.6 kg (8 lb).

The researchers noted that the weight gain they recorded was produced by a limited number of prescription drugs, and that many other drugs that are being prescribed, and which have not been investigated, may also have an effect on weight.

The story went on to suggest that it was perhaps only now, in light of the present epidemic of obesity, that the drugs' negative effect on body weight was beginning to be seen as a problem. In fact, weight gain from prescription medication has always been a problem – albeit one that doctors rarely mention, in part because of the fear that it might make patients less compliant in taking their medication. Indeed, amongst the most frequently asked questions about medications are: 'Is it addictive?' and 'Will it make me fat?'

It is not the obesity epidemic, but the epidemic of pill-popping that has made this devastating (but usually ignored) side-effect much more visible and much more relevant today.

Hard to swallow

While no one knows exactly how many of the currently available prescription drugs can cause weight gain, experts estimate that the list includes more than 50 common medications. To complicate matters, some drugs can cause weight gain in some individuals and weight loss in others. And while some drug-related weight gain can be rapid, it may also take weeks, months or even years to build up, making it difficult to pinpoint medication as the cause. What is more, because so many of us take multiple drugs on a regular basis – more than half of all Americans now take at least one prescription drug, and 10 per cent take at least five different drugs – it can be difficult to decipher which medication (or combination of medications) is interfering with the body's metabolism.

Not all the drugs that we take cause weight gain, but many – which include antidepressants, antipsychotics, birth-control injections, diabetes medications, mood-stabilizers, steroids and medications prescribed for high blood pressure – can do so. Studies show, for example, that one in seven people taking serotonin-enhancing antidepressants like Zoloft and Prozac gain weight. But more than half of those taking the mood-stabilizer Depakote, and three-quarters of patients taking the popular antipsychotic Zyprexa, see their weight shoot up.

More and better research would increase our understanding of the drug/weight-gain phenomenon. Unfortunately, data on body weight is often not recorded in clinical trials, and data on weight gain during drug trials can be obscured by other factors. For instance, if weight loss occurred as a result of illness, weight gain while taking a drug would be considered a benefit, rather than an adverse effect.

What this means is that it is currently impossible to predict who might be more at risk of this kind of weight gain, though certain trends have emerged, thanks to careful studies like that of the Scottish scientists.

How drugs cause weight gain

Just how the majority of drugs lead to weight gain is not well understood. The most common way in which medicines can contribute to weight gain is by increasing the appetite or making people crave certain foods. Some individuals report ravenous hunger while taking serotonin-enhancing antidepressants, antipsychotics and hormones like prednisone and birth-control pills, patches and injections.

The weight gain associated with the use of insulin is thought to be due to the fact that insulin triggers periods of hypogly-caemia (low blood-glucose levels), which in turn stimulate the appetite. Some corticosteroids can make the body less able to absorb blood glucose, and this can lead to fat deposits in the trunk and often significant and swift weight gain. Other medications, such as antihypertensive calcium channel-blockers (which are used to treat high blood pressure), can cause water retention.

Older tricyclic antidepressants (TCAs) and the mood-stabilizer lithium can cause patients to have a dry mouth so that they are more likely to drink high-calorie beverages. Some drugs alter metabolism, causing the body to burn calories more slowly or to store fat. Beta-blockers, which are usually prescribed for high blood pressure, have this effect and can in addition produce fatigue or shortness of breath, making the person less inclined to be active.

For a variety of physiological and psychological reasons, medications can make you tired and thus less motivated to participate in all aspects of life, including exercise. Some drugs – for instance, those that lower cholesterol – can cause or worsen depression, with the knock-on effect that you may feel less motivated to take care of yourself.

While few physicians would care to admit it, many of the medications we take are highly toxic. When the body is exposed to these poisons, it may well react in much the same way as it does when exposed to environmental poisons (see Chapter 4): by trying to dilute the substance, either with fat or by retaining water.

If you are taking regular medication, the weight gain can range from a few pounds to more than 45 kg (100 lb), as can occur with corticosteroids. This excess weight is dangerous because it can cause or worsen problems such as high blood pressure and other cardiovascular conditions, diabetes, high blood cholesterol and osteoarthritis, for which you will then probably be given even more medication.

Drugs that disrupt sleep

Sleep disruption is a major influence on weight gain. A number of prescription medications – especially those that interact with the nervous system – can cause sleep disruption. These include appetite-suppressants, antiemetics, antihistamines, corticosteroids, antihypertensives, diuretics and hormones such as the birth-control pill and HRT, as well as growth and thyroid hormones.

If you are regularly taking these types of drugs, you may be putting on unnecessary weight, due to insufficient or poor-quality sleep (see Chapter 3 for more on sleep deprivation and weight gain).

The worst offenders

A number of studies now show that pharmaceutical drugs used to treat a range of chronic conditions can cause weight gain.[3] These include:

Antibiotics

Antibiotics are overused to an alarming degree in our society. Doctors prescribe them even when they are of uncertain benefit, and patients often demand them for health problems that either won't respond to them (like the common cold) or that will heal just as well over time without them.

But we don't have to be taking antibiotics constantly to be exposed to them. At high doses antibiotics are used to treat infections in animals; at low doses they are used as growth-promoters, causing the animals to gain weight more quickly – and thus command a better price at market.[4] The way antibiotics promote weight gain is by damaging weight-control hormones and interfering with the metabolism.

The use of antibiotics in animals is an ongoing problem, especially in the US and some EU countries. Of all the antibiotics manufactured in the US and the UK, around half are used in livestock. Residues are common in meat and, because we take them in unreasonable quantities too, and because what goes in must come out, there are also antibiotic residues in our water supply.

Antidepressants

In most developed countries, antidepressant use has skyrocketed in the last 15 years. In the UK, for instance, the use of antidepressants increased by 234 per cent in the ten years up to 2002.[5] The number of Britons prescribed antidepressants continues to grow, despite official warnings that many patients may not need them. More than 31 million prescriptions were written by doctors for antidepressant drugs in 2006, with the use of drugs such as Seroxat and Prozac increasing by 10 per cent.[6]

In the US, 11 per cent of women and 5 per cent of men now take antidepressants.[7] According to a recent government study, antidepressants have become the most commonly prescribed drugs in the United States and are now prescribed more than drugs to treat high blood pressure, high cholesterol, asthma or headaches.

In a recent study, the US Centers for Disease Control (CDC) looked at 2.4 billion drugs prescribed in visits to doctors and hospitals in 2005. Of those, 118 million were for anti-depressants.[8] High blood-pressure drugs were the next most-commonly prescribed drug, with 113 million prescriptions. Adult use of antidepressants had almost tripled between the periods 1988–94 and 1999–2000. Between 1995 and 2002 (the most recent year for which statistics are available) the use of these drugs in the US rose 48 per cent.

It is not just adults taking them. The use of antidepressants among US children, for instance, grew three- to tenfold between 1987 and 1996, data from various studies indicate, and a newer survey found a further 50 per cent rise in prescriptions between 1998 and 2002.[9] This explosion in antidepressant use in the US, which is mirrored in the UK and elsewhere, has occurred even though the vast majority of clinical trials have failed to prove that the medicines help depressed children.

Antidepressant use is widely associated with weight gain,[10] and has been since the discovery and use of the first psychotropic drugs. However, the problem has intensified with some of the second-generation antipsychotic medications, such as selective serotonin reuptake inhibitors (SSRIs) like Prozac.

Why this should be so is unclear. Some of these medications might interfere with central-nervous functions regulating energy balance. Some people report an increased appetite for sweet and fatty foods, or 'food cravings' and subsequent weight gain, despite an overall reduced appetite. This may be explained, in part, by the way that some newer antidepressants (TCAs, SSRIs, monoamine oxidase inhibitors or MAO-Is) alter resting metabolic rate.

Antipsychotics

As with antidepressants, the use of antipsychotic medication is on the rise, especially amongst adolescents.[11] Between 1993 and 2003 the number of prescriptions of antipsychotic drugs to children and teenagers in the US increased sixfold. Among the more commonly used second-generation antipsychotic drugs are risperidone (Risperdal), which is used to treat schizophrenia, and olanzapine (Zyprexa), which is used to treat schizophrenia and acute bipolar disorder. However, antipsychotics are also widely prescribed for less clear reasons, such as disruptive behaviour disorders, mood disorders, pervasive developmental disorders and mental retardation.

Most antipsychotics are associated with weight gain.[12] Lithium, in particular, has a marked insulin-like effect, but a number of other antipsychotic medications can increase the risk of impaired glucose tolerance and diabetes mellitus.

Antihypertensives

When a single drug does not sort out a health issue, doctors tend to throw two (or more) at the problem. This is largely how medicine treats the problem of hypertension or high blood pressure. A common combination is a thiazide diuretic (the oldest mainstay of hypertension treatment) combined with a beta-blocker; of the five million people in Britain taking anti-hypertensive drugs, more than one-third take a diuretic/beta-blocker combo.

The problem with doubling up on drugs is the increased potential for adverse effects. When the UK National Institute for Clinical Excellence (NICE) pooled the results of seven studies (involving more than 70,000 patients), it found that the diuretic/beta-blocker combination increased the risk of diabetes by a staggering 20 per cent. Although doctors call this a minimal risk, it represents 6,666 new cases of diabetes every year in the UK.[13] Beta-blockers are also independently associated with weight gain, especially in the first few months of use.[14]

Antidiabetics

Weight gain has been identified as the effect of thiazolidinediones (TZDs) that are widely used to treat diabetes.[15] In placebo-controlled, double-blind clinical studies, increases in average body weight have been observed in people taking TZDs, either as a stand-alone drug or in combination with other antidiabetic agents. Some reviews suggest an average weight gain of 3–4 kg (7–9 lb) over the first six months of TZD treatment,[16] though the rate of weight gain appears to decrease after the first six to 12 months. Other diabetic medications can have the same effect.[17]

For example, in one study after five years of intensive therapy (insulin injections, administered at least three times daily), participants gained 4.6 kg (10 lb) on average compared with those on conventional therapy (insulin injections once or twice a day).[18] Similarly, over ten years in another study, individuals in the intensive blood-glucose control group (taking sulphonylureas or insulin) gained a mean of 2.9 kg (6 lb) compared with those on a more conventional therapy involving dietary changes.[19] Here again a combination of drugs – for instance, TZDs combined with sulphonylureas or insulin[20] – seems to stimulate greater weight gain overall.

Some evidence suggests that antidiabetic medications may contribute to weight gain by triggering the production of new fat cells in certain parts of the body – usually subcutaneous areas such as the buttocks, thighs and lower abdomen.[21]

Steroids

Steroids are hormones. As a broad category of medications, they can include the contraceptive and HRT, as well as the anti-inflammatory medications taken for many conditions including arthritis, eczema and asthma.

All steroids may change the way your body uses sugars and other carbohydrates. Some people temporarily develop diabetes while on steroids. Steroids (including oestrogen[22] and proges-terone) may also cause you to retain salt and fluids, thus making your weight increase. Some, like corticosteroids, also induce potassium loss, which is associated with muscle-wasting (less muscle, slower metabolism).

Birth-control pills can raise insulin levels[23] and lead to insulin resistance, which in turn can raise the risk of weight gain and diabetes. Some may also produce strong cravings. According to anecdotal reports, some women using a trans-dermal (applied to the skin) oestrogen patch report intense hunger, particularly a craving for sweets, whenever it is time for a new patch.

Progesterone increases the appetite and slows down intestinal transit time, thus allowing more of the digested nutrients to be absorbed (good when this hormone is naturally occurring, as it is during pregnancy; not so good if you are eating more for other reasons). It can also sometimes decrease insulin sensitivity, resulting in a degree of insulin resistance that can elevate blood sugar. Progestin, the synthetic form of progesterone found in birth-control pills, can have these same effects.

Similarly, one of the possible adverse effects of corticosteroid use is sometimes massive weight gain, particularly on the trunk and face, as well as fluid retention, a ravenous appetite[24] and uncontrolled hyperglycaemia.

If you suspect that your medication is causing you to gain weight, don't just stop taking it, because this could be dangerous. Instead you should first check the insert that comes with the drugs, to see if weight gain is a reported side-effect. If your weight gain has been rapid – 2.27 kg (5 lb) a month without overeating or underexercising – you may wish to talk with your doctor about changing your medication.

Drugs in the environment

As already hinted at, the problem of exposure to prescription medication is not simply limited to those who actually take these drugs. Few people realize how widespread the problem is, but prescription medications are now ubiquitous pollutants in our environment, especially in our water and food supplies.

Antibiotic residues in animal products account for a large proportion of the pharmaceuticals we ingest each day. Given to animals (including humans) in larger doses, antibiotics are lethal to bacteria. In farming they are used to treat the multiple infections common in industrially raised animals. At low doses, however, these same drugs can cause the animals to gain weight rapidly. Antibiotics can promote weight gain by damaging the hormones involved in weight control and metabolism. Fed to animals surreptitiously and at low doses, these drugs pass into the human food chain, where they can have the same fattening effect in humans.

As far back as 1998 the UK's House of Lords Select Committee on Science and Technology concluded: 'There is a continuing threat to human health from imprudent use of antibiotics in animals.'[25] And in 2001 a report by the Soil Association, the UK's primary organic-certification organization, found that a significant number of chicken samples, including chicken livers, meat and eggs, contained very high levels of synthetic antibiotics known to be damaging to health.[26]

In the EU at least the use of antibiotics as growth-promoters is now being phased out because of concerns about growing antibiotic resistance. But the use of antibiotics as growth-promoters varies wildly throughout the world. Sweden now makes no use of antibiotics for growth-promotion purposes; but the US uses a wide range of antibiotics in all its meat production. Likewise, in Australia a range of growth-promoters is employed.[27] In Brazil – meat supplier to the world's burger bars – antibiotics are used as a matter of routine.

Steroids were used to promote weight gain in farm animals for years (this practice has largely stopped, except in the US, sometimes with startling effects). In one study oestrogens given to chickens made the birds' meat so fatty that it could not be sold.[28]

This means the chances are good that if, like the majority of people, you eat conventionally reared meat – as opposed to organic – you will have ingested metabolically damaging antibiotics at some point in your life.

What's in your water?

Water is one of the most essential nutrients to the human body, ranking second only to oxygen in terms of sustaining life. Humans can't live without water. It is necessary for carrying essential nutrients to the body's cells; it helps transport waste to the kidneys and lungs for excretion; it carries hormones and disease-fighting cells through the bloodstream; it is involved in digestion and metabolism; it regulates our body temperature and our bowels; and it cushions and lubricates our tissues and joints.

To a large extent, our health depends on the quality of the water we drink. And yet drinking a glass of water is increasingly becoming an act of faith.

Any chemical that we use – outside or inside the body – will eventually turn up in our water supply. Although this fact escaped many of us for most of the twentieth century, it was brought into sharp focus in 1971, when the Ralph Nader Study Group in the US reviewed more than 10,000 documents acquired through the Freedom of Information Act. It was able to confirm that US drinking water contained more than 2,100 toxic chemicals that could cause cancer.[29] Things haven't really improved much since then.

The sorts of chemicals most likely to be found in our water include pesticides such as carbamate insecticides (aldicarb and others), the triazine herbicides (atrazine and others) and fertilizers (such as nitrate nitrogen).[30] In addition, our water contains solvents (such as benzene, xylene and trichloroethylene), toxic metals (such as lead, mercury and arsenic) and radionuclides (such as radium). Long-term ingestion of these contaminants has been linked to liver or kidney dysfunction, cancer and reproductive problems.[31] Many of them are also linked to chronic weight gain (see Chapter 4).

Most recently, a new class of water pollutant, composed of pharmaceutical and personal-care products, has been discovered.[32] Pharmaceutical drugs, including antibiotics, hormones, strong painkillers, tranquillizers and chemotherapy chemicals, are now being detected in our surface water, groundwater and drinking water.[33]

German scientists have reported that some 30–60 drugs can be measured in a typical water sample in concentrations similar to those of pesticide contamination.[34] Many of these drugs are specially formulated not to be water-soluble, which means that they will remain intact in our rivers, streams and reservoirs until they are consumed by animals and humans and become stored in the fatty tissues of their bodies.

In 2002 the US Geological Survey (USGS) conducted a landmark study of 139 rivers and streams across the country, and determined that 80 per cent of them contained one or more pharmaceuticals.[35] Then in 2004 the USGS surveyed American waterways in 30 states, testing for 95 different prescription drugs.[36] The survey found that:

- 75 per cent of the water tested contained two or more drugs
- 54 per cent of samples contained more than five drugs
- 34 per cent of samples contained more than ten drugs
- 13 per cent of samples contained more than 20 drugs.

In the UK in 2003 a report by the Environment Agency[37] concluded that the antidepressant Prozac is being taken (and excreted) in such large quantities in the UK that its presence in our water supply was a potential toxic hazard.

We can also be exposed to steroid hormones through the water supply, and this may have effects on our health as well as that of future generations. In animals the administration of steroid hormones during pregnancy can result in offspring having higher weight gain throughout their lives.[38]

Of course, we don't just drink this water – we bathe and shower in it as well, thereby inhaling minute quantities of these chemicals into our lungs. Indeed, it has been suggested that the amount of volatile chemicals inhaled during a 15-minute shower with contaminated water is equivalent to drinking about eight glasses of contaminated water.[39] In addition, many industrial contaminants can easily pass through the skin into the body during showers, baths and dishwashing, more than doubling the amount of chemicals that pass into your body.[40]

Down the drain

There are two primary ways in which drugs get into the water supply:

1 Around half of all the antibiotic drugs manufactured in the UK and the US are fed to livestock. These animals generate significant amounts of manure containing traces of these drugs, which is sold and used as fertilizer on lawns, gardens and farms. When it rains, the drugs in the manure are washed into rivers, streams and underground water supplies.

2 Drugs are flushed down drains and toilets by:
• People cleaning out their medicine cabinets
• Hospitals and drug companies disposing of their old drugs
• People taking drugs and naturally excreting them in human waste.

Many people believe that once they have flushed a drug down the drain or toilet someone else will clean it up. But while water-treatment facilities are equipped to deal with certain types of pollutants, they have no facilities (or remit) to filter out pharmaceuticals that pollute the water supply.

As a result, these substances pass right through sewage- and water-treatment plants into the drinking-water supply. Environmental scientists now believe that these drugs rival pesticides with regard to their contribution to water pollution. Indeed, the 2004 USGS study estimated that the total amount of pharmaceutical and personal-care products released into the environment each year is equivalent to the amount of pesticides released into the environment each year. In the US that is around 400 million kg (888 million lb) of drugs being dumped into the environment – or around 1.3 kg (3 lb) per year for each man, woman and child.

While the disposal of conventional pollutants such as pesticides is regulated, the disposal of drugs is not. Therefore drugs flow unmonitored and continuously into waterways from sewage-treatment plants.

According to an article in the October 2000 issue of the journal *Environmental Health Perspectives*, 'The long-term outcome of humans' ingesting sub-therapeutic doses of numerous drugs as well as any dose at all of substances not meant to be ingested remains a major unaddressed issue.'[41] Either through lack of funding or lack of interest, scientists have not yet conducted the toxicological studies necessary to evaluate the risks posed by chronic exposure to trace concentrations of this cocktail of drugs.

Pharmaceutical apologists maintain that the levels of pharmaceuticals in our drinking water are very low. This may be the case, but it does not make them any less dangerous. If modern environmental science has taught us anything, it is that what is known as 'the low-dose effect' – that is, the impact of minute chronic doses of certain chemicals – can produce some very big effects.

In May of 2007 a team comprising researchers from the Canadian government, the US Environmental Protection Agency and the American Chemistry Council published the results of a seven-year study, during which time the scientists treated an experimental lake in northern Ontario with trace elements of the synthetic hormone used in birth-control pills.[42] For three years between 2001 and 2003 they added synthetic oestrogen to the lake water. The amount used was equivalent to the amount that would be discharged from a city's sewer system. By the end of the experiment, the lake's total concentration of synthetic oestrogen was approximately five parts per trillion, the scientific equivalent of practically nothing. The scientists then watched and waited to see what effect (if any) it would have on populations of the fathead minnow in the lake.

The results were profound. Male fish spontaneously changed sex. They stopped producing sperm and began producing eggs, and their physical appearance changed so that they became indistinguishable from the females. After the first year the minnow population began to decline substantially, and after just a few years the fish were nearly all dead. For the sake of comparison, the scientists also monitored fish populations in two similar-sized lakes in the same area. Fish in those lakes remained completely unaffected, so they could conclude that their oestrogen experiment was the sole cause.

Hormones are not the only harmful drugs in our water supply. Some scientists have also sounded the alarm bell, asking how safe cancer-fighting medicines, which are designed to kill human cells, can possibly be when released into our water supply. Still others have expressed concern that antibiotics excreted by humans into our water may lead disease-causing bacteria to become immune to treatment, which would result in the emergence of drug-resistant diseases.[43]

Such effects are real and measurable. But now we have new concerns to deal with. From the perspective of our ongoing global weight-gain crisis, the release of known obesogenic (obesity-causing) drugs into the environment is now a genuine concern. For years we have been operating under the false hope that once medication goes down the pipes, it is officially somebody else's problem. But, as the evidence shows, drugs in the water have become a problem for all of us.

Cleaner water?

If it's pure water you're after, you may have to create it yourself, using some kind of water filter.

There are several types of water filter, all with differing filtration characteristics and price tags. The simplest is the tabletop jug filter, which usually includes a carbon-based cartridge through which the water is filtered. Other countertop units employ gravity or distillation. You can also buy units that fit directly onto the tap, using a carbon, ceramic or microporous membrane to filter out impurities and provide cleaner water on demand.

Then there is reverse osmosis – a potentially bulky piece of plumbed-in technology. With reverse osmosis, tap water is put through an initial five-micron pre-filter, then a semi-permeable membrane that separates out all the smaller contaminants; 50 per cent of the water is used to flush those away, and the rest is stored as drinking water. The downside is that it is wasteful and removes many beneficial qualities of water, such as minerals, along with the nasty stuff. It is also mildly acidic, which may have long-term adverse health consequences.

Wherever you live, some sort of filtration is probably advisable. But because no filter removes 100 per cent of toxins from the water, we are now in the position where every drink we take – even in the so-called 'civilized' West – has become a compromise.

The illnesses for which we take prescription medications are real – and are another facet of 21st-century illness. So is the largely invisible problem of prescription-drug pollution in our water. As the next chapter shows, there are other invisible influences on weight management lurking in the places that we think are most safe, such as our homes, offices and schools.

CHAPTER 6

The influence of allergies

'Let food be your medicine, and medicine your food.' This is one of the earliest dictats of medical care. Today we know that many of the diseases that plague our modern society have their roots in what we eat, and also in what we don't eat. For instance, a 1997 report by the American Institute of Cancer Research confirmed that between 30 and 40 per cent of all cancers are directly related to our modern diets, which are generally low in complex carbohydrates, fresh fruit and vegetables, and high in fat, salt and additives.

In recent years the field of nutritional medicine, with its emphasis on correcting nutritional imbalance and detecting food sensitivity and allergies, has grown in stature. This is in part because of our increasing awareness that many chronic health conditions can be self-inflicted, sometimes resulting from a combination of unhealthy lifestyles and unfriendly environments. It is also a response to the growing list of adverse effects that accompany the drugs (both prescription and over-the-counter) that we use to suppress the symptoms of chronic illness.

In theory, anyone can be allergic to almost anything. Common substances that trigger an allergic response are dust mites, pollen, pet hairs and bee and wasp venom. Some chemicals, particularly the fragrance chemicals[1] used in perfumes, scented products and air fresheners can also cause allergic reactions. But it is allergies to food and food additives that are arguably the most prevalent type of allergy. As our diets have become much less varied and more loaded with synthetic chemicals, the incidence of food sensitivities of all kinds has increased dramatically, and it is estimated that up to one-third of the population living in industrialized nations has adverse reactions to food.

Food sensitivity can take many forms, the most usual being allergy or intolerance. The two terms are often used interchangeably, but the distinction is important. An allergy is a reaction to a food or other substance that causes an immune-system response. Often (though not always) this response can be measured with immunological blood testing (see page 199). To confuse matters, some experts believe that a person can be allergic to a substance without producing measurable antibodies. Intolerance is a reaction to a food, which does not cause an immune-system reaction (or at least a measurable reaction), but still causes adverse physical symptoms.

Surprisingly there is often little difference in the external physical symptoms, such as skin rashes or respiratory problems – or weight gain – that you may experience, though an allergic response can be much more intense than one caused by intolerance.

When you eat something to which you are allergic, your body reacts as if it has been invaded by an alien organism and marshals all its defences. Your immune system goes on full alert and a series of complex chemical chain reactions take place. Antibodies that fight off the offending substance are produced, and histamine – one of the chemicals that produces symptoms such as breathing difficulties, loose bowels and inflammation – is released. Eventually the toxic by-products of this biochemical war must be excreted from your system, putting your liver and kidneys under increasing strain. Since the skin is one of the major excretory organs of the body, skin rashes can also be the result of the body's attempts to get rid of these toxic by-products.

We still do not know why, for instance, one food or substance should cause an allergic reaction in one individual, but not in another. What we do know is that food sensitivities, including allergies, are a major cause of chronic disease. Over the last few decades the number of allergic reactions that have been identified has grown enormously. There is scientific literature identifying more than 1,700 separate studies that link food sensitivity alone to certain mental symptoms, such as depression and schizophrenia. Clinical papers have also linked food intolerance with Crohn's disease, irritable bowel syndrome, asthma, arthritis, eczema, migraine, hyperactivity and even epilepsy. Many nutritional therapists know this, and the diagnosis of potential allergies is an important part of their treatment.

Despite the accumulating evidence, many conventional doctors are sceptical about the link between allergies and illness. Some are also quick to dispute, often without any real justification, the curative potential of nutritional supplements. So if you suspect that a particular food or something in your environment may be affecting you, it is important to seek the assistance of a qualified nutritional therapist to help you confirm your hunch.

Additives that cause allergies

A raft of synthetic additives contained in modern convenience foods has been implicated in allergic reactions.[2] Reactions to these chemicals can range from a mild upset stomach to severe skin rashes and breathing difficulties. In children some additives, such as colourings and flavourings, have been implicated in behavioural problems.

Flavourings
Aspartame
Monosodium glutamate (MSG)

Preservatives
Benzoates (such as sodium benzoate, potassium benzoate)
Nitrates and nitrites
Sorbates/sorbic acid
Sulphites

Colourings
Amaranth
Annatto
Carmine
Erythrosine
Quinoline yellow
Saffron
Sunset yellow
Tartrazine

Antioxidants
BHA (butylated hydroxyanisole)
BHT (butylated hydroxytoluene)

Emulsifiers and stabilizers

Carrageenan

Guar gum

Gum Arabic

Lecithin

Locust-bean gum

Tragacanth gum

Xanthan gum

Allergies and weight gain

Allergies can produce a variety of symptoms. Some people get skin rashes (atopic dermatitis), some develop asthma and others get allergic rhinitis, or hay fever. Allergies can also reveal themselves through unexplained weight gain.

There are many ways in which allergies can link into overweight and obesity. For instance, one of the problems with a modern diet is lack of variety. Not only is it dull, but over-exposure to the same foods for long periods of time can trigger allergic symptoms. Studies show that many overweight patients have an increased hypersensitivity to foods. These sensitivities can in turn trigger a reduced ability to metabolize fats. Thus food allergies may be playing a key role in temporary weight gain as well as in long-term obesity.

An allergy can cause the body to retain a surprising amount of excess fluid (see box on page 128). The allergic reaction itself can also produce a drastic reduction in blood sugar (hypoglycaemia), with the accompanying symptoms of weakness, hunger and irritability. This reaction usually occurs two to six hours after ingesting the offending food, and can be severe enough to stimulate persistent hunger and trigger the unhealthy eating patterns that are often implicated in the development of obesity.

Allergic hunger is pathological inasmuch as it does not respond to the normal satiety control centre in the brain when food is consumed in normal amounts, so both the cravings and the allergic symptoms caused by allergies can cause uncontrollable eating behaviour. In addition, many medications used to treat allergy symptoms often trigger weight gain as a side-effect, without ever addressing the actual cause of the immune response.

Allergy and addiction

Food sensitivities may cause people to crave those foods to which they are allergic. Just as a drug addict suffers withdrawal symptoms when the drug is withdrawn, so allergic people experience discomfort when they stop eating (or lose access to) a particular food.

The phenomenon of simultaneous allergy and addiction to both foods and chemicals is now well accepted by doctors specializing in the diagnosis and treatment of allergies. It can, however, be difficult to trace the offending food, because over time the allergy can become 'hidden'.

In the allergy-addiction cycle there are three principal stages: the first is characterized by an acute allergic reaction to a substance the body perceives as toxic. A good illustration of this is when someone first inhales a cigarette. Frequently that first puff will taste terrible and will even produce symptoms like coughing, sore throat and dizziness – signs that the body has identified the cigarette smoke as poisonous. But after smoking becomes a habit, these symptoms are no longer noticeable. The body's natural reaction becomes masked, or hidden, as it tries to adapt to a poison with which it comes into frequent contact.

The next stage is when adaptation turns to addiction, so that you must smoke regularly to avoid withdrawal symptoms. All addictions – to cigarettes, coffee, heroin, wheat or milk products – are similar in this regard. If this cycle goes on long enough, the body begins to produce symptoms of chronic poisoning.

Many overweight and obese people are all too aware of the overwhelming power of food-allergy addiction. Compulsive eaters crave, and continue to eat, those allergenic foods to which they are addicted – even though they feel worse and not better after eating them.

This phenomenon has been widely researched. Some scientists speculate that frequent contact with allergenic foods triggers a rise in the brain-chemical opioid enkephalin. The enkephalin is a narcotic produced by the body that is as addictive as externally supplied narcotics.

According to Charles E. Bates, author of *Beyond Dieting: Relief from Persistent Hunger*,[3] delayed (or non-IgE) food allergy may be at the root of obsessive eating habits. He believes that obesity may be a symptom of an immune mediated eating disorder (IMED), which is caused by a combination of digestive-system and immune-system errors that arise when we continue to eat foods to which we are allergic.

This process of errors is cumulative, says Bates, and may begin in infancy. Signs of IMED are apparent in babies who have feeding problems, colic or some kind of chronic indigestion, diarrhoea, allergies, eczema and an inability to tolerate certain foods such as cow's milk. Later they may show a tendency towards chronic bronchitis and middle-ear infections. In school they may show signs of learning disabilities or hyperactive behaviour. By adulthood there may be more complaints: irritability, joint pain, noticeable fatigue, depression and migraine, gastritis, ulcers and heartburn. Any chronic inflammatory disease of the upper or lower gastrointestinal tract is also a significant sign of an allergy of some type.

Allergies and 'water weight'

An allergic reaction to food may cause the body to retain as much as 4 per cent of its body weight as oedema (excess water in the body tissues).[4] Thus a sudden weight gain, possibly signalled by such signs as increased thirst and swelling of feet and hands (resulting in 'tight rings' or 'tight shoes'), may be an important indicator of an undiagnosed food allergy. The removal of an offending food will often result in a rapid water loss of 2.2–4.5 kg (5–10 lb) within a week's time, all without the use of a diuretic.

Allergy specialists have observed this water-retention phenomenon frequently among patients, and comment anecdotally that once the offending foods are removed from the diet and the patient has dropped a significant amount of water weight, that person will then go on to lose fat more easily, even without restrictive dieting.

Bates's theory sits well with other theories about the potential link between blood type and diet.[5] While not well researched, the theory goes that dietary lectins (specialized proteins found in grains, beans, dairy products and certain vegetables) can trigger different allergic responses in different individuals, depending on their blood type.[6] If lectins pass undigested into the gastrointestinal tract, they are either recognized as self or non-self by the body's immune system. Cooking breaks down and eliminates a significant percentage of dietary lectins, but not all. Some, such as those present in wheat, tomato, carrot, corn, banana, peanuts, pumpkin seeds and avocado, are highly heat-resistant.

Although not specifically centred on obesity, the research into blood type and diet shows that certain blood groups react badly to certain types of foods, resulting in allergies, inflammation and leaky gut, as well as gut disorders such as Crohn's disease. It is the link with inflammation that may be the most important where allergic weight gain is concerned.

Allergies and inflammation

When you are exposed to or ingest something to which you are allergic, your body reacts as if it is under attack and this is a stress response. One of the first symptoms to be produced is inflammation. Inflammation is primarily a protective measure. Most of us are familiar with it. If you bang your thumb with a hammer or skin your knee, or a cut becomes infected, the tissues around the injury swell up, and this acute inflammation is a quick response that protects the injured area by surrounding it with extra padding and a rich supply of blood to help it heal.

But exposure to small amounts of daily poisons can also produce chronic inflammation – a more subtle condition that is now being linked to a raft of health problems that develop over the longer term, such as heart disease, respiratory illness and cancer. Most recently chronic inflammation has also been linked to obesity. The reason is that chronic inflammation can set up a resistance to the weight-management hormone leptin (see pages 32–35). This in turn can produce a sluggish metabolism and sometimes overwhelming cravings. Weight gain or loss in the face of inflammation is not a matter of will or discipline, but of a chemical imbalance. Correct the chemical imbalance and the weight will begin to come off.

Chronic inflammation, sometimes called silent inflammation, is a modern condition. It can be caused by a poor diet,[7] by a sedentary lifestyle,[8] by unchecked stress[9] and by environmental toxins.[10] On their own, each of these factors produces a kind of low-grade inflammation in the body. Combined, they can produce substantial effects. A body with chronic inflammation is a chemically altered body. It is awash with inflammatory chemicals trying to protect the body and with anti-inflammatory chemicals trying to counterbalance them.[11] It is the anti-inflammatory chemicals that appear to disrupt the body's natural response to leptin.

Some physicians such as Dr Leo Galland, author and internationally recognized expert in nutrition, believe that industrial pollutants can also cause allergies and allergic responses that can create, or worsen, the problem of chronic systemic inflammation.

According to Galland,[12] who has been studying and working with the effects of chronic inflammation for years, fat produces leptin in order to regulate itself. These increased levels of leptin should speed up your metabolism; however, chronic inflammation disrupts this process, triggering leptin resistance.

For Dr Galland, it is the problem of chronic inflammation that is most relevant to rising levels of obesity. Inflammation, he argues, causes the body to release a range of chemicals that make the system resistant to the relatively recently discovered hormone, leptin.

Inflammation can cause obesity, but obesity can also cause inflammation,[13] resulting in an endless feedback loop of ill health. Obesity can raise levels of hormones known as adipokines, which set off the body's inflammatory response. The more body fat you have, the more adipokines you will produce. These hormones are responsible for some of the diseases that are linked to obesity. TNF-alpha (tumour necrosis factor alpha), for example, is known for producing the tissue damage associated with rheumatoid arthritis and other autoimmune conditions. TNF-alpha also interferes with the body's response to insulin and is thus a major contributor to insulin resistance.[14] Another adipokine, interleukin 6 (IL6), is associated with arthritis and heart disease.

Fat also attracts a type of white blood cell known as a macrophage.[15] Macrophages are scavengers; their job in the body is to clean up cellular debris, especially in and around fat cells. Once inside the fat call, macrophages also produce inflammatory chemicals and this output is met by the fat cell producing a range of anti-inflammatory chemicals as a counterbalance. These anti-inflammatory substances are known as suppressors of cytokine signalling (SOCS). SOCS also interfere with leptin by disabling the signal that tells the body to speed up metabolism and suppress appetite.[16]

Allergies and obesity/overweight is a vicious cycle that can be made worse if your diet is high in foods that also produce inflammation. This includes allergens such as food additives and colourings, as well as refined sugars, trans fats and red meat.

According to Galland, the science is difficult, and yet some understanding of it is crucial if we are to get to grips with the problems of hard-to-shift weight. 'Whenever there is inflammation, the cells respond by producing anti-inflammatory chemicals known as SOCS – suppressors of cytokine signalling. Two of these, SOCS1 and SOCS3, interfere with leptin by blocking the signal in the cells,' he comments.

The mechanism is very similar to the development of insulin resistance, which is also due to inflammation. In fact, inflammation also causes production of the 'fight-or-flight' hormone cortisol from the adrenal glands. Cortisol blocks leptin and it also raises blood sugar which in turn decreases the response to any given amount of insulin.[17]

The bigger picture of what he is saying is staggering. Inflammation is fundamentally a protective process that is necessary, for instance, for wound-healing as well as for curing infection. If inflammation arises in a polluted body, it is highly likely that it is a protective response to the presence of allergens and/or toxins.

How is inflammation measured?

Doctors can get an idea of the level of inflammation in your body by measuring a substance known as C-reactive protein (CRP). In particular CRP is a good indicator of levels of interleukin 6 (IL6) in the bloodstream. As weight goes up, levels of CRP go up too, and elevated levels of CRP are associated with a higher risk of certain obesity-related diseases, such as high blood pressure[18] and heart disease.[19]

Testing for allergies

Identifying and eliminating allergies can sometimes be harder than it sounds. Someone who suspects they have a food allergy may find resistance from their medical practitioner, and as a result may find it hard to get the testing they need. The tests themselves – while becoming more and more accurate – may only detect the most gross allergic reactions.

The classic biological marker for an allergy is an antibody called IgE (immunoglobulin type E). When the offending food enters the bloodstream, the body produces IgE antibodies for that food. These antibodies trigger the release of chemicals, including histamine, that cause the classic symptoms of allergy: skin rashes, hay fever, rhinitis, sinusitis, asthma, eczema, swelling in the face or throat. All of these 'IgE-mediated' reactions are immediate and severe, and can even be life-threatening, as in the case of anaphylaxis (an acute allergic reaction). If you have this type of allergy, you probably already know about it and do all you can to stay away from the offending food.

The more common type of food allergy, however, involves a different marker called immunoglobulin type G (IgG). The difference is that IgG reactions may take anywhere from an hour to three days to show themselves, are often less immediately dramatic in nature and are therefore much harder to detect. This makes it more likely that you will be continuing to eat foods to which you are allergic on a regular basis, without making a connection between your symptoms and the offending food.

According to Allergy UK, around one in four of the population will at some time in their lives see a doctor because of an allergy. Allergy testing is therefore becoming increasingly sophisticated. The type of test you may be subjected to will depend upon your symptoms and the condition of your skin.

With allergy testing, doctors are looking for measurable reactions to food, such as the presence of IgE and IgG antibodies. Skin-prick or scratch tests measure IgE reactions on the skin. This is usually the first test that is recommended when an allergy is suspected. It is simple, quick (you get the results within 15–20 minutes) and inexpensive. But, for reasons that we do not yet fully understand, skin-prick testing with food allergens is less reliable than with other allergens such as fungus spores, pollen, house dust mites, animal hair and so on, and so false negative reactions (where you are told you are not allergic, even though you are) can occur.

Patch tests – where a bandage with specific allergens is left on the skin for several hours – also search for IgE responses and are usually performed on eczema patients suspected of having an allergy. Blood tests like the Allergen-Specific IgE Antibody Test (RAST) also measure the amount of specific IgE in circulation. Blood tests may sometimes indicate an allergy, but not which food is linked to any symptoms, nor can they predict the severity of any food reaction.

Simple food-sensitivity tests usually look for one group of antibodies, the IgG4 group. However, newer lab tests, such as the Enzyme-Linked Immunosorbent Assay (ELISA) or tests looking for the whole range of IgG (1, 2, 3 and 4), are supposed to make the process more accurate.

In the main, allergy testing cannot tell you about food 'intolerances' – where your body, say, lacks some enzyme and cannot cope properly with the corresponding food. This means that more subtle, subclinical intolerances that do not register on standard tests may go undetected and continue to wreak havoc in the body.

There is, however, another fly in the ointment – and this applies to all types of nutritional and allergy analysis. The quality of the laboratory that performs the test is crucial to getting an accurate result. Recent evidence suggests that laboratories can vary widely in terms of sample preparation methods and calibration standards.[20] Not all these things are easily controlled by the consumer/patient – but it is as well to be aware of them and to choose your practitioner carefully.

Allergy testing can be expensive and, even with increasingly sophisticated technology at our disposal, is not always accurate. Elimination regimes – overseen by a qualified nutritional therapist or allergy specialist – are thus still the best way to detect and deal with allergens. On such a regime the person is placed on a very simple diet that eliminates all potential allergens. These foods are then introduced back into the diet one at a time, to judge whether or not the person reacts to them.

Dealing with cravings

Food cravings and aversions are a normal part of life. While aversions can be difficult to explain, cravings have come under much scrutiny over the years. Often the craving is not for the food itself, but for what it contains and the effect it has on your body. Equally, a craving can be the result of a dietary imbalance; diets that are high in grains often produce wild cravings in some individuals. A craving is not a bad thing – it is a message from your body.

If you are in tune enough, you will be able to respond to it appropriately. If a craving is allowed to turn into a binge, however, it can exacerbate existing imbalances. Most of us find it easy to give in to cravings for chocolate and other sweet treats, but too much sugar is certainly not good for you and can drastically reduce your immune response. This is just one reason why it may be helpful to try and understand where cravings come from and the best ways to deal with them.

Annemarie Colbin, American nutritionist and founder of the Institute for Food and Health in New York, combines Western and Eastern perspectives in her work. Over the years she has identified three main reasons for cravings:

• Addiction and allergy are two sides of the same coin. They both produce psychological or physiological symptoms that can be temporarily suppressed by eating the longed-for food. Eating the food makes the person feel better, though it does not cure the underlying problem.

• Discharge is the term for a person who has changed their diet and is experiencing a longing for a food that is no longer part of their regime. When you alter your diet – for instance, changing from a diet high in processed foods to a raw food diet – the body begins to release, or discharge, toxins as well as the chemical 'memory' of these foods. The body may interpret this chemical memory as need, even though it is not a genuine craving. That is why, when you do eat the longed-for food, it isn't as satisfying as it might be.

• Imbalance is another very common problem created by modern diets. In a fast-moving world we tend to grab quick foods, and often our diets are very high in one particular sort of food (usually carbohydrates) at the expense of others. Since the primary aim of the body is equilibrium, a craving for a particular food or foods can be seen as the body's attempt to restore balance. In particular, a craving for fats and sweets together, such as those contained in baked goods and ice creams, may be a signal of protein deficiency.

Dealing with cravings

Craving	Consider	Eat more
Sugar (for example, cakes, pastries, cookies, sweets and ice cream)	Restrict your intake or eliminate it completely	Whole grains, baked yams, squash, apples, dates, cooked fruit
Salt	Limiting your intake	Seaweed, black beans, vegetables
Milk products	Cutting down or eliminating them completely	Leafy greens, whole grains, beans, fish
Fats and sweets (including baked goods made with natural sweeteners, wholewheat flour and oils)	Limiting your intake	Proteins such as beans, fish, chicken, eggs
Coffee	Cutting it out of your diet	Vegetables, salad
Alcohol	Cut down or eliminate it completely	Complex carbohydrates, vegetables, corn, leafy bitter greens

To diminish or eliminate a craving, use the information in the chart below, which is adapted from Colbin's excellent book, *Food and Healing:*[21]

In addition, American nutritionist Earl Mindell[22] believes that the common cravings in the chart on page 138 may signal the need for an increase in specific nutrients.

Eat less	Try instead
Meat, salt, dairy	Frozen bananas instead of ice cream; desserts sweetened with barley rice syrup and maple syrup
Sweets, fats, alcohol, meat, grains	Natural soy sauce, miso (in small amounts), herbs and spices
Sugar, baked goods, fruit, meat	Tofu (in small amounts), nut milk
Grains, fruit, salad	None
Salt, acid-forming foods such as meat, sugar, flour, grain	Grain coffee, herbal teas
Fats, salt, miso, soy sauce, animal protein	Non-alcoholic beer, fruit juices, herb teas

Common cravings for vital vitamins

Craving	Nutrients required
Peanut butter/nuts	B vitamins, protein and fat. A good-quality supplement will help diminish the craving and will be lower in calories
Olives, pickles	Sodium, necessary for the proper functioning of nerves and muscles and for water balance; but too much can cause hypertension
Bananas	Potassium, which helps to maintain the body's water balance and normalize the heart beat
Cheese	Calcium, phosphorus and aluminium; eat more broccoli as a lower-fat alternative
Apples	Calcium, magnesium, phosphorus, potassium; in addition, if you have a high-fat diet, your body may be craving the pectin for its ability to lower cholesterol
Cantaloupe	Potassium and vitamin A are its main nutrients, but it also contains vitamin C, calcium, magnesium, phosphorus, biotin and inositol – so it's not a bad craving to give in to
Milk	Calcium is the obvious choice, but milk also contains useful amino acids such as tryptophan, leucine and lysine; as long as you're not allergic, have the odd glass
Eggs	Full of protein, but also sulphur, amino acids, selenium and, in the yolk, fat; the white, by the way, contains useful fat, dissolving choline, which is why the humble egg is considered a first-class protein meal

Finally, some people – women in particular – experience uncontrollable cravings for chocolate. Chocolate is a complex food, the consumption of which begins a complex series of biochemical reactions in the body. Cravings for chocolate need to be addressed on both the physical and emotional levels. Eating chocolate may stimulate the release of 'feel-good' brain chemicals (called neurotransmitters) in the body; this, combined with the immediate sugar boost, may help a woman who is tired or depressed to feel better, albeit for a short time.

Most commercially produced chocolate, however, is laced with pesticides, additives and other undesirable synthetic chemicals (most of which are not listed on the label). A more positive approach to feeling good would be to pursue a regular course of exercise and relaxation and, if necessary, consult a therapist to deal with feelings of depression and lack of self-worth. Chocolate also contains magnesium and iron, so another tactic is to make sure that you are getting enough of these nutrients through your daily diet.

Tackling food allergies – or allergies of any kind – can require a detective's attention to detail and the patience of a saint. However, for many people who find their weight hard to shift, it can make shedding the pounds much easier in the long run. Allergies, like all the other influences on weight that are described in this book, place the body under tremendous stress. As the next chapter reveals, stress can have its own devastating effect on your metabolism.

CHAPTER 7

The stress factor

The experience of feeling stressed is a fact of modern life. The frayed nerves, the short temper, the anxiety, depression and fatigue that make up the emotional experience of stress are all too familiar in our day-to-day lives.

In our cave-dweller past, our bodily responses to severely stressful situations – increased blood pressure and pulse, respiratory rate, energy requirements, muscle tone and perspiration, all triggered by the release of stress hormones – kept us safe when under attack from wild animals or warring tribes. These 'fight-or-flight' responses have been exquisitely honed over the lengthy course of human evolution. Their purpose was to preserve life by providing a keener perception of potential dangers, greater strength in combat or other physical challenges, and greater speed, enabling escape from potentially dangerous situations.

Because of the flood of stress hormones that gets released when we are under stress, a body under stress is a chemically altered body. It is a body awash in hormones and other substances that are normally kept under tight control. In the right proportions hormones such as catecholamines (including dopamine, epinephrine and norepinephrine), glucocortoids such as cortisol, and androgens such as dehydroepiandosterone (DHEA) keep our bodies healthy.

But get too much or too little of them and they become a form of slow poison, leading to a simply staggering list of stress-related disorders. This list now includes fatigue, indigestion, infections, irritability, diarrhoea, eczema, headaches, constipation, psoriasis, muscle tension, peptic ulcers, allergies, neck and back pain, irritable bowel syndrome, asthma, atherosclerosis, nutritional deficiencies, high blood pressure, anorexia nervosa, premenstrual symptoms, diabetes, sexual problems, arthritis, insomnia, psychological problems, cancer, depression and weight changes. Indeed, no part of our lives remains untouched by stress.

The human body is a vastly complex organism. It is finely tuned and adaptable. Indeed, it is this ability to adapt that helps us maintain our normal physiological state of balance. Our fight-or-flight responses are part of an inbuilt survival mechanism. Through a process referred to by doctors as 'allostasis'[1] – the ability to achieve harmony and balance through change and adaptation – your body is constantly adjusting itself to the prevailing conditions. The problem is that a body that is constantly adjusting itself to stressors is subject to a great deal of wear and tear. With all this overactivity, the adaptive mechanisms become worn out, leading to an inability to either adapt or shut themselves off (thereby reducing the levels of circulating stress hormones) once the stressful event has been resolved.[2]

The complex relationship between physical and psychological health is still not well understood. But we do know that the major body systems – nervous, endocrine and immune – are intricately linked. They share hormones, neurotransmitters and cytokines (substances that promote cell growth and division), a relationship that helps maintain the equilibrium necessary for a healthy body. However, in times of stress, one or more of these systems may be affected, and what disrupts the balance in one system can disrupt the others. The interactions between these systems have given rise to an entirely new branch of medicine: psychoneuroimmunoendocrinology. Study in this field has greatly enhanced our understanding of the intricate workings of the body.

Through allostasis two adaptive pathways – the hypothalamic-pituitary-adrenal (HPA) axis and the sympatho-adrenal-medullary (SAM) axis, which controls the sympathetic nervous system – are initiated. Activation of these pathways leads to many neuroendocrine changes, such as an elevation in hormones and proteins – for example, cortisol, epinephrine, norepinephrine, calcitonin, gastrin and insulin – which can result in common fight-or-flight responses like elevated blood pressure, heart and sweat rate, coagulation (blood-clotting) time and blood-glucose levels.

During episodes of acute stress, hormones such as cortisol at first protect us by activating the body's defences through a complex chain of biochemical events. But when these same protective hormones are released repeatedly or in excess, as in the case of chronic stress, they can cause a gradual and steady cascade of harmful physiological changes. As levels of cortisol rise in response to chronic stress, so levels of another hormone, DHEA, drop. The result can be hypothyroidism (underactive thyroid), heart disease, prostate and breast cancer, menstrual irregularities, osteoporosis and autoimmune disorders such as systemic lupus erythematosus (SLE) and rheumatoid arthritis.[3]

What is more, as part of what is known as a 'general adaptive syndrome', we become less and less sensitive first to whatever is stressing us, and second to the chemicals that our body released in order to help us cope. So in the same way that diabetics can become insensitive to the high levels of insulin released into the bloodstream to cope with excess glucose, and the bodies of people who are continually subject to toxic chemicals and allergens adapt to a chronic poison (see Chapter 6), so the bodies of people under stress become less and less sensitive to the increasing amounts of cortisol released into their systems.

Stress, whatever its origin, can also become a circular path. For instance, physical stress can lead to emotional stress, and vice versa. In addition, it is not just major stressors that cause problems. Evidence shows that high numbers of small daily hassles can take their toll.[4] But whatever the source and intensity, the body responds if it is under attack by releasing a flood of stress hormones to help it maintain balance. When this happens the usual recommendations, such as relaxation and exercise, may no longer be enough to counteract the effects of stress.

Stressed-out pets

Our pets can suffer from all the same disorders that we suffer from, including, it seems, the effects of stress. A recent survey for UK pet insurer More Than showed that obesity and behavioural symptoms are significantly on the increase as the health of the nation's pets is in decline.[5]

The survey, comprising 100 vets and 2,500 owners, found that almost 80 per cent of vets were seeing more obese pets, and blamed the animals' obesity on a lack of exercise, overfeeding and poor diet. A quarter of pets suffer from stress, hyperactivity and depression, while three-fifths of vets claim that even more are suffering from diabetes and arthritis.

Even when faced with an obviously overweight pet, the study claims, around 90 per cent of owners still refuse to believe that their pets are overweight.

A body awash in stress hormones for years at a time is most likely to develop a range of diseases and declines in mental and physical functioning, all of which modern physicians consider common with advancing age.

For instance, a lifetime of job stress (which usually involves high psychological demands and a perceived lack of control) can accelerate the progression of atherosclerosis and heart failure.[6] Caring for a spouse or relative who is ill, for example with Alzheimer's disease, can also lead to a greater risk of coronary heart disease.[7]

Higher cortisol levels have been recorded in patients with heart disease.[8] Stress can also raise blood pressure,[9] create harmful free-radicals (rogue molecules that attack body tissues and cause degeneration) and raise levels of homocysteine (an amino acid that damages cell linings and artery walls).[10]

An eight-year study of 73,000 people in Japan recently showed that women who reported high mental stress were more than twice as likely to have a fatal stroke than those reporting low stress, and about three times as likely to have a deadly heart attack. Men who reported high mental stress were about one and a half times more likely to die from a heart attack, though they did not show significantly increased deaths overall from strokes.[11]

Although the women who reported high stress were more sedentary, more likely to have a history of hypertension or diabetes, smoked more and were more likely to work full time, the researchers concluded that, even after adjusting for these factors, the association between stress and heart attacks in both women and men, and an association between stress and strokes in women, remained.

Stress and weight gain

In developed countries where life tends to be competitive, fast-paced, demanding and stressful, new links are continually being drawn between so-called modern life and increasing rates of overeating, overweight and obesity.

Chronic stress appears to feed both indirectly and directly into weight gain, through the way it alters our moods as well as the way it disrupts levels of key hormones. Stress alters the levels of several key brain hormones and may therefore lead to a lack of impulse control (and thus control of overeating habits). It is also associated with bad nutritional habits, like unpredictable eating times and eating much more rapidly than normal, or eating until you feel uncomfortably full. Given all this, it is hardly surprising that stress has been shown to lead to poor eating habits, poor glucose control and eventually obesity[12] – cornerstones of many diseases later in life.

Two hormones, epinephrine and norepinephrine, released when you are under stress, trigger the fight-or-flight response. A third hormone cortisol, provides the energy for this response by stimulating insulin release and rapid fat and carbohydrate metabolism. This increases a person's appetite for high-starch and high-fat foods. If you are under constant stress, your cortisol levels will remain elevated. With elevated cortisol, people often turn to 'comfort food' – such as breads, pastas, sweets and high-fat snacks – for relief. Indulging in such foods is not just a psychological response; it is also a response to high levels of fight-or-flight chemicals circulating in the body.[13]

Stress also inhibits the release of serotonin, a neurotransmitter that affects appetite, mood, learning and memory. Carbohydrates help increase serotonin levels, producing a calming affect.

The way in which stress stimulates an appetite for comfort foods was highlighted recently in animal research from the University of California at San Francisco, published in the *Proceedings of the National Academy of Sciences*. In order to investigate the biological link between stress and the drive to eat, Professor Mary Dallman and her colleagues[14] simulated chronic stress by increasing the brain concentration of a rodent version of cortisol. As concentrations of this stress hormone rose, the rats responded by drinking increasingly more sugar water, eating increasingly more lard – and gaining abdominal girth. The researchers noted that comfort foods that were high in sugar, fat and calories appeared to calm the body's response to chronic stress.

Stress, memory and mood

Stress does more than poison the physical body. It also has a profound effect on our minds and moods. The same hypothalamic-pituitary-adrenal (HPA) activity that causes physical disorders in some people can cause mental and emotional disorders in others. Long-term stress may also affect memory by destroying neurons in the hippocampus, the area of the brain that contributes to visual memory and context.[15]

The poor dietary habits associated with stress may also contribute to a range of psychological problems, including mild depression and anxiety.[16] Depressed individuals often have significantly higher morning and midnight salivary cortisol levels[17] and disrupted circadian rhythms – that is to say, the natural 24-hour rhythms of sleep and waking.[18] At the extreme end of the scale, about some 60 per cent of chronic schizophrenia patients also show abnormal cortisol levels.[19]

Women in particular are more prone to a depression/obesity cycle. Depression can both cause and result from stress, which may in turn cause women to change their eating and activity habits. In one study, obesity in women was associated with a 37 per cent increase in major depression. Another study of obese people with binge-eating problems found that 51 per cent also had a history of major depression.

The link with stress and depression is important because depressed individuals may be less inclined to take care of themselves and to make positive nutritional choices. They may also fall prey to compulsive eating habits.

In addition, hormones such as cortisol also encourage the formation of fat cells.[20] And to add insult to injury, research has found that high cortisol levels are linked to a tendency to store excess fat in the abdomen (rather than in the hips, thighs and buttocks).[21] Excess abdominal fat is particularly dangerous as it places a greater strain on the heart and is associated with an increased risk of cancer and diabetes. Even healthy-weight individuals who are 'high-stress responders' have been found to store extra abdominal fat.

Indeed, a theory known as the 'stress cascade' suggests an interconnection between stress, glucose metabolism, obesity, hypertension and altered fat metabolism[22] – all of which are aspects of the Metabolic Syndrome (see page 59).

The stress cascade results in the release of increasingly large amounts of catecholamines and corticosteroids, which in turn affect insulin regulation, glucose metabolism and fat storage. Sustained cortisol output caused by stress increases insulin insensitivity, tending to lead to decreased tissue glucose uptake. When this happens, insulin levels rise to counteract the increasing insensitivity to insulin.

Long-term elevations of cortisol along with the increase in insulin also increase the accumulation of visceral fatty tissue – for instance, around the abdomen – creating a much higher risk of heart disease and diabetes as we age.

Sadly, children are not immune to the stress/weight-gain cycle. A good example of this effect has recently come from doctors at Bristol University in the UK.[23] Girls in the UK are reaching puberty one and a half years before their mothers did, and two years before their grandmothers did. The onset of puberty in the UK now starts when a girl is ten years and three months old, and it seems that the trend towards earlier puberty is advancing.

The Bristol scientists found a possible explanation in the appetite-controlling hormone, leptin, which is produced exclusively by fat cells (see pages 32–25). Girls in the UK are heavier than they used to be. Because they are carrying more fat, they are also producing more leptin. This overproduction of leptin may be interfereing with their levels of reproductive hormones, specifically progesterone and oestrogen. This, combined with an increasingly stressful life, which further alters hormone levels, may be triggering earlier and earlier menstruation.

Can stress be good for you?

The right kind of stress may actually be beneficial.

Investigators now distinguish between passive stress (for instance, watching a scary movie) and active stress (such as trying to meet a deadline). According to one report,[24] active stress can boost the immune system, increasing one's ability to fight off infection.

The researchers evaluated 30 male volunteers who were exposed to two different types of stressful situations: an 'active' stressful event, where volunteers were asked to memorize information and take a 12-minute test; and a 'passive' event, where volunteers watched a 12-minute video of 'gruesome' surgical procedures.

During the experiments each person gave saliva samples that were analysed for immune-system components known as secretory proteins. These proteins help protect the lining of organs such as the lungs and stomach, guarding against the invasion of bacteria and viruses. While levels of secretory proteins increased during active stress, the immune response actually dropped during passive stress.

Most acute stressors boost the immune system, at least initially. It is only when stress is unusually prolonged or repetitive that it becomes a potential threat to health. An exception to this rule appears to be when we experience stressors for which the only response is to endure passively. These types of stressors, over which we feel we have no control, have a rapid and strong suppressive effect on some aspects of immune function.

Bungee-jumpers, parachutists and other thrill-seekers will be delighted to hear that the authors of this study recommend these kinds of challenges as being active and beneficial to the immune system and thus to your overall health.

Environmental stress

Most of us continue to equate stress with the physical and emotional experiences of everyday life, although today these are more likely to concern bereavement, marriage, divorce, long working days, a new baby and unemployment rather than encounters with wild animals. But as humans have evolved, other sorts of stressors – physical, chemical, electromagnetic, nutritional, traumatic and even psychospiritual – have come into play. On a chemical level, the body does not differentiate between emotional stress and environmental stress. Anything that threatens to unbalance or harm the body can trigger its primitive fight-or-flight responses and cause the release of a flood of stress hormones (see Chapter 4 for more on environmental pollution and weight gain).

Most of us are unaware of the contribution of environmental factors – for instance, exposure to pollutants, pharmaceutical drugs and noise pollution – to our stress levels. And yet, because they tend to bypass our conscious awareness, environmental and other stressors that are not emotional or psychological in nature are arguably the most harmful to our health.

When speaking of toxic exposures, the effects of stress should not be underestimated. A stressed-out body is a body less able to deal with poisons in the environment. It is one that may, ultimately, become overwhelmed and less efficient at metabolizing and excreting toxins. When your internal systems are not working to excrete toxins, the body tends to limit the damage by 'diluting' toxins. It does this in one of two ways: by retaining water or, if the toxins are fat-soluble, by storing them in fat. Not surprisingly, puffiness and weight gain, which are in themselves physically and emotionally stressful, are also associated with a body that is overwhelmed by toxic pollutants.

Certainly, in the face of the insidious poison of environmental hormones and indoor air infused with harmful gases, which surrounds us each day, the usual behavioural solutions for managing stress – such as reframing your perceptions of that stress to make them more positive or sharpening your coping skills – aren't really effective. After all, there isn't anything inherently positive about being poisoned. In a body overwhelmed by environmental poisons, usually effective recommendations such as relaxation and exercise (see below) may no longer be enough to counteract completely the effects of stress.

Few of us have the choice of living in an unpolluted environment. City dwellers are often obliged to travel and live in places where pollution from cars and factories is a fact of life. Many of us work and live in buildings so full of chemicals that they have come to be known as 'sick buildings'. Good evidence shows that many of the substances that we come into contact with each day are causing a health crisis in our bodies, and it behoves us to do what we can to reduce our exposure, whenever and wherever we can.

How to beat stress

At some point in their lives virtually everyone will experience stressful events or situations that overwhelm their natural coping mechanisms. People respond to stress differently depending on different factors, such as early nurturing, personality traits, genetic factors, immune-regulated diseases and the length and intensity of stressors.

Nevertheless studies indicate that the following people are more vulnerable to the effects of stress than others. The very young and the very old, for instance, can be prone to stress-related illness, though stress often goes unnoticed in these age groups. Others at risk include:

• Women in general, but particularly working mothers
• Less-educated individuals
• Divorced or widowed individuals
• The unemployed
• Isolated individuals
• People who are targets of racial or sexual discrimination
• City dwellers.

How we perceive and manage stress is important to our overall health. When stress becomes too great, the damage may be irreversible. So to maintain and even improve your level of health, start taking action now.

• Exercise. Of all the things we can do to lower stress levels and counteract the allostatic load, exercise – along with a prudent diet – seems to be the most effective. Moderate exercise (defined by the National Institutes of Health as roughly equivalent to physical activity that uses about 150 calories of energy per day, or 1,000 calories per week) helps improve sugar metabolism through the more efficient use of insulin, and assists in ending the vicious cycles of stress-eating, overindulging in alcohol, cigarette smoking and other unhealthy habits.

• Consider adaptogenic herbs. Adaptogens work on a cellular level to normalize the function of every cell, thereby stimulating the healing process to enhance the body's natural defences and helping the body to function normally. Adaptogens have been found to provide temporary relief from the symptoms of many conditions that are brought on by stress. The major ones include schizandra berries, astragalus, ashwaganda, reishi mushrooms, gotu kola, holy basil, Angelica sinensis (dong quai), echinacea, royal jelly and – perhaps the most well-known – ginseng (Korean and Siberian). If you are at all unsure what to take, consult a qualified herbalist.

• Consider better nutrition ... Nutrients commonly depleted by stress include the antioxidant vitamins A, E and C, as well as vitamin B-complex and the minerals zinc, selenium, calcium, magnesium, iron, potassium, sulphur and molybdenum. Along with a wholefood diet and a high potency multivitamin and mineral supplement, ensure that you get adequate levels of B-complex and vitamin C. B vitamins are necessary to protect the brain and nervous system; B6 (20–50 mg daily) can alleviate depression, and B12 (1,000 mcg daily) is necessary to maintain a healthy nervous system. Similarly vitamin C is a valuable anti-stress antioxidant – aim for 500–1,000 mg daily. Among the minerals, calcium (500–750 mg daily) and magnesium (350–500 mg daily) should be considered. Many of these nutrients are also necessary for an efficient metabolism.

• Avoid alcohol. A high intake of alcohol may blunt the body's ability to respond appropriately to stress. People who abuse alcohol have all kinds of health-related problems and often find adapting to stress difficult – a problem related to worn-out adaptive pathways.[25]

• Try stress management – it can make a difference. Stress-management techniques address the behavioural aspect of 'handling' stress. People with heart disease can lower their risk of subsequent cardiac events by more than 70 per cent if they learn how to manage stress.[26] Similarly, stress-management techniques have been shown to improve glucose control in diabetics.[27] Stress management can take the form of formal behavioural modification or of new/old practices such as yoga and tai chi.

• Quit smoking. Habitual smokers have higher cortisol levels following cigarette smoking compared to non-smokers. Ironically, smokers can exhibit lower cortisol levels than non-smokers when challenged by a psychological stress, though this is probably due to lowered HPA response.[28]

• Stay optimistic. Two recent studies[29] have found that optimists live longer and better. Optimists tend to develop better coping skills and a more supportive social network than those with a darker outlook, and this may shelter them from stress, illness and depression.

• Hug your children and teach them to cope better than you have. Experts have found that being touched and held during the first few years of childhood may set up positive stress-response patterns that last a lifetime.

To cope with personal, social and environmental stress, you need to be aware of your lifestyle and your environment, and understand how these things can affect you, even when you are not immediately aware of these effects. Once you know the sources of your environmental stress, the only way to 'cope' is to remove as much of it as possible from your life. Doing so will pave the way for the dietary changes suggested in the next chapter, which can help your body burn calories more efficiently.

CHAPTER 8

You are what you eat

If diets don't work and you want to lose weight, what else can you do?

Most experts agree that the most successful long-term weight-loss programmes encompass more than just keeping an eye on calories. A multidimensional approach to healthy eating requires a long-term commitment to changing your habits and ingrained ideas about food and to opening up to a much more holistic concept of health. Such an approach will generally:

• Strongly discourage dieting

• Foster the idea that all foods are okay, within moderation

• Encourage greater attention to signals of hunger and satiety – in other words, to eat when you are hungry and stop when you feel satisfied

• Encourage awareness of when you are eating to fulfil emotional needs rather than physical ones, or as a means of coping with stress

• Provide alternative ways to meet emotional needs and to respond to stress in a more constructive way.

This kind of approach is the antithesis of the single-dimensional quick-fix mentality. Indeed, a healthy approach to weight loss requires you to take on several important conceptual changes.

Most people are encouraged to lose weight because they are dissatisfied with themselves. It is this dissatisfaction that makes you vulnerable to the seduction of the quick fix. Undertaking a commitment to lose weight from a perspective of acceptance – even love – puts a whole new spin on the project and provides a much more positive platform from which to change your eating habits, and indeed your entire lifestyle.

For people whose daily lives have been bombarded with images of physical perfection, and who have come to believe that they must be a certain shape or size to be attractive or loved or accepted by others, self-acceptance may be the hardest perspective to attain. Yet knowing yourself and your body from many perspectives, enjoying your strengths and beauties, whilst objectively and dispassionately being aware of your limitations and weaknesses, can be enormously liberating. It can make the task of changing your lifestyle much more rewarding.

Another important concept, closely allied to self-acceptance, is acceptance of the idea that what constitutes a 'healthy weight' is much more flexible and inclusive than most of us realize. In the spectrum between anorexic and obese there is a large and healthy area in which most of us can comfortably live. At least we can if we are prepared to give up two things: a) unreasonable ideas about quick weight loss; and b) freakish ideas about what men, women and especially children are supposed to look like.

From the perspective of this book, another type of acceptance is also required for steady weight loss: acceptance that the world has changed – largely due to our own carelessness; that the hallmark of the 21st century is a toxic environment that is damaging to all living systems, including that of the human body. It is not just a polluted physical environment that we live in, but a toxic emotional and psychological environment that we have allowed to predominate as well. Exposure to the 'stress' of modern life, as this book has shown, is as polluting and toxic as exposure to poisonous chemicals.

Because we are sensitive, complex beings, we respond to our environments. So if you want to lose weight, it may be that a significant step forward is to 'lose' those aspects of modern life that are making that goal difficult to achieve. Thus, in addition to the general concepts already outlined, a multidimensional approach to weight loss would include getting a good night's sleep, removing allergens and (as far as possible) environmental toxins from your life, making relaxation a priority, avoiding unnecessary drugs and, where possible, discussing with your doctor ways of cutting down on your use of medication.

Each of the preceding chapters has offered advice on how to deal with these 21st-century influences on weight gain. What hasn't yet been addressed in depth is what we do eat, or should be eating, in order to stay healthy.

'Bad' food

There is diversity of opinion as to whether it is appropriate to give too much focus to the quality of food intake and whether it is helpful to talk to dieters in terms of 'good' and 'bad' foods. Some nutritionists believe that overweight and obese people have been so besieged by dietary advice that attention to these matters would feel like a perpetuation of restriction and would interfere with the ability to take on board new ideas.

Others believe that food intake impacts on health and well-being to such a significant degree that we must all be more attentive to the nature of the food we select. In fact, many suggest that some of the health impairments experienced by some obese persons are the result of poor food intake resulting from years of selecting foods on the basis of what would promote weight loss, rather than what is healthy. These nutritionists advocate an attitude of taking individual responsibility for the quality of your intake, just as you take responsibility for your dental care or the use of seat belts.

Using absolute terms like 'good food' and 'bad food' is probably not helpful, and yet it is also true that food can be 'bad' for you in lots of ways. You can eat too much of it and become obese (a major risk factor for heart disease, stroke and diabetes, among other things). It can contain pesticides, contaminants and 'anti-nutrients' (substances that prevent the body absorbing essential nutrients, such as soya flour). Or it can contain so few nutrients that you 'starve', even when you appear to be eating plenty.

Each of these problems is linked. For instance, when you eat nutrient-poor food, your body doesn't get all it needs to stay healthy. It instinctively knows this and craves more and more food in order to get what it needs. When you give in to these cravings and continue to eat calorie-rich, nutritionally poor foods, you gain weight. The more excess weight you carry, the more capacity you have for storing things like pesticides and other synthetic chemicals in your body. The more chemicals in your body, the greater the risk of declining health.

Food fads have also drastically altered the way we eat. Most of us have a list of 'good' and 'bad' foods informed by the cult of food 'experts' who offer advice in newspapers, books and magazines that subtly inform our food choices. Much of the constantly changing advice of dieticians and government bodies – reduce fat, eat raw foods, follow a 'Mediterranean diet' – has never been researched in detail, and some of it is downright damaging. In fact it has been said that you have a better chance of winning the lottery than you have of hitting on clear and accurate advice about what you should be eating.

Humans thrive on variety, yet diet-faddists encourage us to cut out specific types of foods, even entire food groups, from our daily diet in order to be 'healthy'. At the same time market forces encourage us to consume a whole range of novel convenience foods – often in great quantity – that may not be good for us and may not even be food in any real sense of the word.

Indeed, much of what we call food today would only have existed in the realms of science fiction one hundred years ago: exotic items grown without soil, flown in daily from far away, made from ingredients synthesized in the lab and preserved long beyond their natural shelf life with a variety of industrial chemicals derived from petroleum by-products.

We eat meat by-products enhanced with artificial meat flavours to make them palatable. We eat processed, quick-cook microwave and oven meals. Even the so-called 'healthy' cereals that we eat for breakfast are so highly processed and nutritionally poor that the manufacturers have to add vitamins to them, simply so that they can be classified as foods.

Every day we put this nutritionally impoverished, adulterated, unbalanced stuff into our bodies and, when our bodies eventually stop functioning properly, we wonder why. The fact is that our daily diets are the most influential aspect of our day-to-day health. What we eat is reflected in the strength of our immune and hormonal systems, the way our minds function, our muscle coordination, the health of our bones, the quality of our skin and hair, the short- and long-term health of the children we produce; and the health problems associated with consuming a poor diet – heart disease, cancer, arthritis, diabetes and obesity – are real and tangible.

What can you do?

The rules of healthy eating are familiar to most of us, and yet how many of us manage to follow them?

• Eat when you are hungry, stop when you are full (or maybe a little bit before).

• Eat slowly, and savour your food. This is a much more pleasurable thing to do – and a much easier thing to do – if the food you are eating is fresh and flavourful. Snack foods, which don't have the complex favours of natural foods, are designed to be eaten quickly. Eating good food slowly is a sensual pleasure and gives your body a chance to signal to you that it has had enough; this will cut out your chances of overeating.

• Practise portion control. What we consider a normal portion has almost doubled in the last few decades. It is always better to start off with less on your plate, eat slowly and then decide if you need more. Many of us could comfortably cut the volume on our plates by half and still be adequately nourished (and still include small indulgences from time to time).

• You don't need to eat three full meals a day. For some people, eating smaller, more frequent meals works better to stimulate their metabolism. Try eating no more than three hours apart if you are a woman, or five hours if you are a man (male metabolism is slower) and see if it works for you.

• You *do* need to eat breakfast. The time between eating dinner and eating breakfast is probably the longest that any of us go without food during any 24 hours. Everyone needs a top-up meal in the morning to revive flagging energy and sustain them through the day.

• Make greens one of the staples of your diet. Eat plenty of fruit and drink diluted pure fruit juice or water.

• Include more complex carbohydrates, including wholewheat bread, wholemeal pasta, potatoes, brown rice, millet, oats and rye, as another of the staples of your diet. Avoid refined carbo-hydrates – any 'white' sugars or cereals in general – as well as chocolate, sweets, biscuits, pastries and soft drinks.

• Think of meat and dairy as condiments, rather than mainstays of your diet. We all need protein, but in general we all get far too much of it. Reducing the quantity of meat and dairy you consume means that you can opt to buy better-quality, organic options, which will help reduce your exposure to unwanted agricultural chemicals.

• Ditch the convenience-food habit. Convenience foods are low in nutrients, foster poor eating habits and usually contain refined carbohydrates, sugar and high levels of fat and salt.

• Develop the habit of reading labels carefully. Choose foods with the shortest list of ingredients, ideally all organic whole foods.

• Reduce (and preferably avoid) stimulants, including tea, coffee, chocolate, tobacco and canned drinks that contain caffeine. Substitute them with herbal teas, grain coffee, spring water and diluted pure juices. Avoid decaffeinated coffee, which still contains other stimulants.

• Avoid foods that have been hydrogenated, which create trans fats that are stored as fat.

• If you need something sweet, try fruit – fresh or dried. Use maple syrup, honey, concentrated apple juice, barley malt and date syrup as substitutes for refined sugars.

• Reduce your intake of salt, which retains water. Salt also masks the natural taste of food and is probably only necessary when food is of poor quality. Buy the best, freshest food you can and relearn to appreciate its natural flavour.

Polluted food

Even when we try to eat 'good' foods there are hidden dangers. Health professionals recommend that you eat at least five servings of fruit and vegetables every day as part of a varied diet. Unfortunately, if you eat conventionally grown produce, you may also unknowingly be ingesting a mixture of harmful pesticides, including:

• Insecticides to control insects
• Rodenticides to control rodents
• Herbicides to control weeds
• Fungicides to control mould and fungus
• Antimicrobials to control bacteria.

Many of these, as outlined in Chapter 4, can interfere with the body's natural weight-management systems. Just because you can't see or taste them doesn't mean they aren't there. The most comprehensive testing for the presence of unwanted chemicals in food is the ongoing US Total Diet Study (TDS), conducted by the US Food and Drug Administration (FDA) and updated yearly. The TDS looks for the presence of many different chemicals in food, but its findings on levels of chlorinated pesticides have been particularly distressing. In its 1988 report, DDE (a close relative of DDT) was found in every single sample of raisins, spinach (fresh and frozen), chilli con carne (beef and beans) and beef.[1]

DDE was also found in 93 per cent of processed cheese, mince, hot dogs, collards (spring greens), chicken, turkey and ice-cream wafer-sandwiches sampled. It was also present in 87 per cent of lamb chops, salami, canned spinach, meatloaf and butter, and in 81 per cent of sauces and creamed spinach.

Since DDT and DDE have been banned in the US since 1972, it is likely that some of this contamination is from produce imported from other countries that still use these chemicals. But some of it is also because of the persistence of these chemicals in the soil; growing crops or rearing animals on land contaminated with DDT and DDE means that we 'recycle' these toxins back into the food chain.

In the intervening years, things haven't got much better. The 1999 TDS showed that, among the foods sampled, 17 different pesticides were found in butter, 32 in cherries, 29 in strawberries and 27 in apples.[2] The baked-potato samples contained 23 pesticides and hamburgers 22; milk-chocolate samples contained 18. Once again, DDE/DDT was the residue most often found, with chlorpyrifos-methyl, malathion, endosulfan, dieldrin and chlorpyrifos also being very common.

In the UK the 1999 Annual Report by the Working Party on Pesticide Residues (WPPR) found that 27 per cent of the full range of foods tested had pesticide residues. Among them, DDT (which is banned in the UK) was found in beef slices, corned beef and lamb's kidney; and the herbicide 2,4-dichlorophenoxyacetic acid (2,4-D) (also banned in the UK) was found in more than half the oranges tested. Oranges, pears, lettuces, chocolate and apples contained the highest numbers and levels of residues.[3] Three-quarters of the chocolate samples contained lindane (a relative of DDT), and one in eight jars of baby food was also contaminated. Surveys in Australia and New Zealand have found similarly high levels of pesticides in foods.[4]

Government surveys around the world continue to show that consuming many everyday staple foods, such as fruit, vegetables, cereals, bread, dairy products, meat and fish, as well as wine and beer, can increase our exposure to this cocktail of chemicals exponentially.

We are what they eat

In recent decades our consumption of meat products has grown dramatically. In the West the average person eats around 62 kg (137 lb) of beef, chicken, fish and shellfish per year. If you eat meat, then you are also eating whatever the animal ate before it was slaughtered.

There was a time when animals reared as food ate what grew naturally: cows and chickens ate grass and grain; big fish ate small fish or other sea creatures. In industrialized meat production – often a 30,000-cow feedlot or a 60,000-chicken coop – things are very different. The artificial conditions in which the animals are kept (often minus light and regular exercise) and the requirement for the animals to grow quickly to a saleable weight means that they require special 'scientific' diets. Such facilities need huge quantities of high-protein rations, and this has coincided with the need for slaughterhouses to find a cheap, safe way to dispose of waste. Both industries have entered into a marriage of convenience, which means that a number of animal by-products are now included in animal feed – even for those animals that are not natural carnivores.

Cattle and chickens are still given plant-based feed: corn (for carbohydrates) and soybean meal (for amino acids) make up 70–90 per cent of most commercial animal feed. But the remaining 10–30 per cent can differ radically from what cows and poultry would eat in their natural habitat.

Processed feathers, for instance, are an acceptable source of protein in cattle feed, as are chicken faeces. Plastic pellets are permitted as roughage. Chickens can be fed meat and bone meal. And in addition to their main diet of fishmeal and fish oil, farmed fish may be given rendered meat, bone and feather meal. These animal by-products can be contaminated with bacteria such as salmonella, and the recycling of animal by-products into animal feed is also considered a risk for mad-cow disease.

Other animal-feed additives contain worrying industrial toxins. Every year in the US 5 billion kg (11 billion lb) of animal fat is recycled into animal feed – worrying, since many toxins and pesticides such as dioxins and PCBs concentrate naturally in animal fat. Dioxins also concentrate in the clays that occasionally get mixed into animal feeds.

Also included in the food of intensively reared animals are medications such as growth-promoters and antibiotics, which are given routinely – even to healthy cattle and chickens – to hasten growth and keep infections at bay. There is growing concern about the high use of antibiotics and the possible effects on human health. Antimicrobial drug residues in food (including antibiotics) are suspected of causing allergies, cancer, paralysis and respiratory failure, anaphylactic shock and aplastic anaemia in either humans or animals. Antibiotics are also used as growth-promoters in animals because, even at low doses, they cause animals to gain weight quickly. If you are ingesting meat products that contain antibiotics, they may be contributing to the problem of hard-to-lose extra pounds.

Finally, every time we ingest antibiotics in our meat we are contributing to the worldwide problem of antibiotic resistance. Nevertheless the default position of many government committees is that these residues pose no risk to consumers.

Little is known about the effects of multiple pesticide residues: the cocktail effect. There has been very little research done, but all current knowledge points to the distinct possibility that chemicals would react with each other to form even more potent toxins.

Officials continue to argue that levels of pesticide residues in food are within legal limits, but until this is proven safe beyond all reasonable doubt, we should not allow ourselves to be lulled into a false sense of security – 'legal' does not necessarily mean 'safe'.

What can you do?

Once they are on or in food, pesticides are very difficult to avoid. Some authorities recommend that we wash and scrub all fresh fruit and vegetables thoroughly under running water. Running water has an abrasive effect that soaking does not have, which may help to remove traces of chemicals from the surface of fruit and vegetables and dirt from the crevices. But not all pesticide residues can be removed by washing because many are designed to be water-resistant – and thus not to wash off crops when it rains.

Peeling the skin of fruit and vegetables when possible, and discarding the outer leaves of leafy vegetables, can reduce your exposure. So can trimming the fat from meat and skin from poultry and fish, because most pesticides residues collect in fat.

Eating a variety of foods is also sometimes recommended to help reduce your exposure to any single pesticide. It is uncertain how effective this is, because most pesticides function in similar ways and, on the journey from farm to table, many foods are coated with multiple pesticides and fungicides. From a health standpoint, however, eating food from a variety of sources will give you a more comprehensive mix of nutrients and this may have a protective effect.

In fact the best – and probably the only – way to avoid pesticides in your food is to include as much organic food in your diet as possible. While the price of organic food is coming down each year, it can still be so expensive that it is beyond some people's food budgets. This doesn't mean that you need to be resigned to a refrigerator full of toxic food. One way to lower your burden is to prioritize, reserving organic purchases for those foods known to contain high levels of pesticides and other toxins, such as dairy and meat products and grains.

The level of pesticides in fruit and vegetables can vary enormously, depending on the crop and the season. Research in this area has revealed some startling findings. In 1995 the Environmental Working Group (EWG), a pressure group based in Washington, DC, reviewed studies conducted by the Food and Drug Administration and the Environmental Protection Agency into the pesticide contents of 42 different types of produce in the US.[5] They found that some types of produce had very little pesticide residue. According to their findings, the least-polluted products (in ascending order to the most polluted) were:

• Avocados
• Corn
• Onions
• Sweet potatoes
• Cauliflower
• Brussels sprouts
• Grapes (US)
• Bananas
• Plums
• Spring onions
• Watermelon
• Broccoli.

But, among the most contaminated, there were a few surprises. Strawberries were contaminated with more types of pesticides than any other fruit or vegetable, followed by peppers, spinach, cherries, peaches, celery, cantaloupe melon, apples, apricots, grapes, green beans and cucumbers. Pesticide residues cannot easily be washed off and are often absorbed into the flesh of the plant, so even peeling the skin of certain fruits will not reduce your pesticide intake by much. Instead, as the chart below shows, the EWG recommended that, if you regularly eat these foods, you should consider substituting other foods of equal or better nutritional value and lower pesticide rating.

EWG suggested food alternatives

Food	Main nutrients	Alternatives
Strawberries	Vitamin C	Blueberries, raspberries, blackberries, oranges, grapefruit, cantaloupe, kiwis or watermelon
Peppers	Red peppers contain carotenoids (vitamin A),and both green and red peppers are rich in vitamin C	Alternatives to green peppers: green peas, broccoli or romaine lettuce; alternatives to red peppers: romaine lettuce, carrots, broccoli, Brussels sprouts, asparagus or tomatoes
Spinach	Carotenoids (vitamin A), vitamin C and folic acid	Broccoli, Brussels sprouts, romaine lettuce or asparagus
Cherries	Vitamin C	Oranges, blueberries, raspberries, blackberries, grapefruit, cantaloupe or kiwis
Peaches	Carotenoids (vitamin A) and vitamin C	Nectarines, cantaloupe, watermelon, tangerines, oranges, red or pink grapefruit

Cantaloupe	Carotenoids (vitamin A), vitamin C and potassium	Cantaloupe in season (May–December) or watermelon
Celery	Some carotenoids (vitamin A), but not a good source of vitamins	Carrots, romaine lettuce, broccoli or radish
Apples	Vitamin C	Pears, oranges, grapefruit, cantaloupe, kiwis, watermelon, nectarines, bananas, tangerines or virtually any fruit not on the 'most contaminated foods' list
Apricots	Carotenoids (vitamin A), vitamin C and potassium	Nectarines, cantaloupe, watermelon, tangerines, oranges, red or pink grapefruit or watermelon
Green beans	Not a particularly rich source of vitamins or carotenoids	Green peas, broccoli, cauliflower, Brussels sprouts, potatoes or asparagus
Grapes (Chilean)	Vitamin C	Grapes in season (May–December)
Cucumbers	Not a particularly rich source of vitamins or carotenoids	Carrots, romaine lettuce, broccoli, radish or virtually any vegetable not on the 'most contaminated foods' list

The benefit of eating lots of fruit and vegetables – especially if they are fresh and from local sources – generally outweighs any potential risks from low-level pesticide residues found in produce. Nevertheless, why voluntarily ingest high levels of pesticides when good alternatives are available, either through buying organic or by choosing your non-organic produce (and other foodstuffs) carefully?

Missing nutrients

Apart from the things that are added intentionally or otherwise to our food supply, there are a whole host of things that we have lost, due to modern intensive agriculture. These also have important implications for our long-term health and weight maintenance, since adequate vitamins and minerals are necessary to maintain a healthy metabolism.

While fruit, vegetables and whole grains are commonly thought to be high in essential nutrients, the majority of today's produce and grains are grown in depleted soil, doused with pesticides and stored for long periods of time (all the while being sprayed with more insecticides and fungicides) before being sold. They may be stored for an even longer time after purchase before being eaten or used in cooking.

Because of this, some modern nutritionists believe that, in the midst of all this plenty, many people in the West are starving – for the basic nutrients that were once in our everyday food.

Conventional farmers are caught in a vicious circle of production. They add chemical fertilizers to the soil in the hope of increasing crop yields, but doing this ultimately increases many plants' susceptibility to pests. So more pesticides are used. But the pesticides they use can also affect the soil's capacity to sustain and generate fertility.

Using synthetic fertilizers to make plants grow in otherwise depleted soils has other disturbing consequences. For instance, while the fertilizer will stimulate the plant to grow, in the absence of any of the usual protective nutrients they should contain, the plants will also take up more of the heavy metals in the soil, such as aluminium, mercury and lead, and these, in turn, are passed on up through the food chain. All the while, the nutritional value of our food is plummeting.[6]

In 1940 British chemists Robert McCance and Elsie Widdowson published the first of what would be their periodical examinations of the nutrient content of food.[7] When the fifth edition of this tome – which has over the years become a standard reference work on the subject – was published in 1991, a British geologist-turned-nutritionist, David Thomas, undertook the work of comparing the values as published in the first and last editions of the book.[8]

He examined the data for 28 raw vegetables and 44 cooked vegetables, 17 fruits and ten types of meat, poultry and game, and his findings make frightening reading. What he found was that, amongst today's foods:

• Potatoes have 30 per cent less magnesium, 35 per cent less calcium, 45 per cent less iron and 47 per cent less copper
• Carrots have 75 per cent less magnesium, 48 per cent less calcium, 46 per cent less iron and 75 per cent less copper
• Broccoli (boiled) has 75 per cent less calcium
• Spinach (boiled) has 60 per cent less iron and 96 per cent less copper
• Swedes have 71 per cent less iron
• Spring onions have 74 per cent less calcium
• Watercress has 93 per cent less copper
• All meats contain 41 per cent less calcium and 54 per cent less iron
• All fruits contain 27 per cent less zinc

• Apples and oranges have 67 per cent less iron.

Among other worrying findings was that seeding the soil with only certain minerals (sodium, phosphorus and potassium) has greatly altered the natural mineral profile of our foods. Thus, swedes now contain 110 per cent of the phosphorus they once did. Humans who eat this nutritionally altered food cannot help but experience an alteration in the natural mineral profiles of their body tissues and bones as well.

A similar exercise was carried out in the US in 1999 when nutritionist Alex Jack compared nutrient values in the current US Department of Agriculture (USDA) handbook with those published in 1975.[9] He discovered a number of mineral deficits, as well as the fact that cauliflower had 40 per cent less vitamin C than it did in 1975.

Many classes of herbicide can alter plant metabolism and, therefore, nutrient composition. For example, herbicides that inhibit photosynthesis (such as triazine or phenoxyacetics) produce effects similar to growing a plant in low-light conditions. Under such conditions, the carbohydrate, alpha-tocopherol (vitamin E) and beta-carotene (a precursor of vitamin A) content of a plant is reduced, and protein, free amino-acid and nitrate levels are increased. Equally, bleaching herbicides can reduce beta-carotene levels, and sulphonylurea herbicides are known to reduce levels of branched-chain amino acids (which humans need in order to maintain muscle tissue).

What can you do?

In a perfect world, nutritional supplements would not be necessary. We would get all the nutrients we need from our diet. But this is not a perfect world and the combination of nutrient-poor food, everyday pollutants and stress can deplete our bodies of what they need in order to function well. Although they are not panaceas, nutritional supplements can help to make up for some of the deficiencies in your diet. While you are normalizing your weight, you may need to take some in amounts that are higher than the RDA (recommended daily amount), which is the minimum amount that most of us need in order to stave off severe deficiencies.

As detailed in the early chapters of this book, body fat acts like a storage system for toxins.[10] Dr Elson Haas, director of the Preventative Medicine Center of Marin County in San Rafael, California, believes that obesity is almost always associated with toxicity and that any weight-loss regime should include measures to support the body as toxic chemicals are released.[11] When we lose weight, we reduce our fat and thereby our toxic load. But during weight loss we also liberate more of these toxins and thus need more protection. While losing weight, greater intakes of water, fibre and antioxidant nutrients such as vitamins C and E, selenium and zinc – as well as liver-support herbs such as milk thistle – may be appropriate means of protection. If you are at all unsure about what to take, consult a qualified nutritionist.

Below is a brief list of some of the best nutrients for boosting metabolism, fighting toxic exposure and keeping free-radicals under control, and maintaining a healthy immune function. Supplements should not be taken in isolation, since many nutrients rely on the presence of others to work well. When you are taking 'extra' supplements, it is helpful to take a basic multivitamin and mineral tablet as a foundation.

Glutathione

Glutathione is a sulphur-containing amino acid found in high concentrations in liver cells. Studies have shown that glutathione attaches to toxic compounds in the liver, neutralizing them or enabling them to be excreted.[12] Glutathione is too large a molecule to effectively pass through the intestine into cells, so supplementing with glutathione alone is not helpful.[13] But when taken with vitamin C, which protects it from oxidative damage, glutathione is recycled and becomes effective.[14] A useful amount is 1 g daily, though some people may benefit from 2–3 g daily.

Vitamin B-complex

B vitamins help to optimize metabolism and are important for the transportation of energy in the body. A good B-complex supplement should contain a minimum of 50 mg of each of the main B vitamins, including B_1 (thiamine), B_2 (riboflavin) and B_6 (pyridoxine).

Vitamin C

Vitamin C, or ascorbic acid, aids the detoxification process in several ways. In the same way that it recycles glutathione, it also recycles other antioxidants, including vitamin E, making them more effective. Aim for 1 g daily.

Vitamin D

In the days before the sun became our enemy, we got all the vitamin D we needed by exposing ourselves regularly to the sun. Today a largely unjustified fear of skin cancer has meant that we shun the sun. Studies show that we need adequate vitamin D in order to lose weight.[15] Vitamin D is, in addition, anti-inflammatory and immune-enhancing.[16] Most of us need 400–800 units of vitamin D daily taken with a meal.[17] To help your body produce vitamin D naturally, try – where possible – to get at least 15 minutes a day of exposure to the sun (without sunblock) on your hands, arms, face and legs.

Vitamin E

The major fat-soluble antioxidant in the body, vitamin E is the most-studied free-radical quencher.[18] Vitamin E and water-soluble vitamin C work synergistically in the fight against free-radicals. Vitamins C and E, as well as beta-carotene, protect the liver from damage and help to support detoxification mechanisms.[19] Vitamin E is believed to be non-toxic even in high doses, but most of us need only supplement with 400–800 iu (international units) each day.

Calcium

Research suggests that low calcium intake can stimulate the production of body fat and interfere with its breakdown.[20] Try taking calcium citrate in doses from 500 to 1,000 mg daily.

Magnesium

Adequate intake of magnesium can aid sleep and muscle relaxation. If you are stressed or exercising hard, or are exposed to environmental toxins or allergies, supplements can help. Aim for 100–300 mg per day.

Zinc

This is an important antioxidant and helps to keep the liver functioning well. Adequate zinc can boost immunity, protect against free-radical damage, maintain healthy cells and help guard against copper overload. A great many people do not get enough zinc. A reasonable daily supplement would be 25–50 mg.

Selenium

Selenium is essential for proper immune function and may have anticancer effects.[21] It also helps to make zinc more effective, and works closely with vitamin E to maintain not just a healthy liver, but a healthy heart as well. Animal studies have found that selenium from yeast is better absorbed than selenium in the form of selenite.[22] Taking 200–300 iu daily is considered healthy.

Can fats make you thin?

Forget your fat phobia. Increasing your intake of healthy fats is important to maintaining good health. Good fats can help leach toxins out of your system, prevent inflammation and reset your natural weight-management systems.

In general, there are two main 'families' of essential fatty acids (EFAs): omega-6 and omega-3. In each family of EFAs there is a particularly important acid: in the omega-6 family it is linoleic acid (LA). This is converted in the body to gamma-linolenic acid (GLA) and later into the series 1 and 2 prostaglandins that, in high quantities, can have a deleterious effect on health.

In the omega-3 family, alpha-linolenic acid (LNA) is the most important. In the body this is converted to eicosapentaenoic acid (EPA). EPA can also be synthesized in the body from docosahexaenoic acid (DHA). EPA and DHA help keep our arteries clean and our platelets less sticky. EPA is the starting material for making series 3 prostaglandins, which have beneficial effects on blood pressure, cholesterol and blood-fat levels, as well as kidney function, the inflammatory response and immune function. Too much or too little of these prostaglandins can leave the body unable to cope with illness.

Generally speaking, we get far too much omega-6s and not nearly enough omega-3s. In a healthy diet the ratio of omega-6 to omega-3 should be 2:1.

According to fats expert Udo Erasmus,[23] including more of these healthy fats in our diet while avoiding trans fats may encourage the body to lose weight (a good way to also lose stored toxins). In his experience, those who take 45–70 ml of mixed omega-3 and omega-6 fatty acids (the equivalent of 3–5 American-sized tablespoons, 4–7 UK dessertspoons or 2–3 UK tablespoons) will consistently lose weight even if they don't alter their diets. He adds, however, that the results will be better if the EFAs are part of a comprehensive diet regime that includes increasing your intake of greens, cutting down on saturated fats, switching to organic foods wherever possible and supplementing with digestive enzymes.

To get your daily dose of good fats, British nutritionist Patrick Holford suggests the following:[24]

The best natural sources of omega-3
• LNA: flaxseed, hempseed, canola, soya-bean and walnut oils, and dark-green leaves
• EPA/DHA: cold-water fish, salmon, mackerel, sardines.

You can get what you need from
• Hempseed oil, 1 tablespoon
• Flaxseed oil, 1 tablespoon
• Flax seeds, 2 tablespoons
• Pumpkin seeds, 4 tablespoons
• EPA/DHA supplement, 1,000 mg.

The best natural sources of omega-6
• LA: safflower, sunflower, hemp, soya bean, walnut, pumpkin, sesame and flax
• GLA: borage seed, blackcurrant seed, evening primrose oil.

You can get what you need from

- Hemp seeds, 1 tablespoon
- Sunflower seeds, 1 tablespoon
- Pumpkin seeds, 2 tablespoons
- Sesame seeds, 1.5 tablespoons
- Evening primrose oil, 1,000 mg
- Borage oil, 500 mg.

Choose one source of omega-3 and omega-6 from each list to achieve a good intake of EFAs. Another good source of both types of fatty acids is dried beans, such as kidney, haricot and chickpeas. Regularly including these in your diet will ensure that your EFA needs are met.

How should we be eating?

The more we learn about the toxic potential of modern foods, the greater the need for a new food culture that values wholesomeness, nutrition, freshness and flavour. Raising our expectations of food and embracing these values has the knock-on effect of protecting the natural environment, treating animals humanely, protecting our soil and respecting the farmers and food-industry workers who are involved in the food-production process. It also leads to a stronger preference for foods that are produced locally. If you are ready to take that responsibility, then getting back to good food is probably much easier than you think. You can choose, for instance, any or all of the following ways to improve your daily diet.

Eat local

When it comes to eating good food, most of us would automatically think organic. Organic food has undoubted advantages, but in the big picture of food production, locally produced food has a much more important role to play in keeping our bodies and communities healthy.

Consider the conclusions of a 2005 study by British researchers, published in the journal *Food Policy*.[25] The team calculated a shopping basket's hidden costs, which mount up as produce is transported over large distances. The study found that 'road miles' account for proportionately more environmental damage than 'air miles'. While organic farming is valuable, the miles that organic food often travels to reach our plate creates environmental damage that outweighs the benefit of buying organic.

Instead, they argued that people can help the environment even more by buying food from within a 20 km (12 mile) radius. By their calculations, if all foods were sourced from within 20 km of where they were consumed, environmental and congestion costs would fall from more than £2.3 billion to under £230 million – an 'environmental saving' of £2.1 billion annually.

Buying locally produced food might seem impossible if you live in a big city. But by patronizing farmers markets or making use of delivery schemes you can drastically cut your contribution to food miles and put fresher, better food on your table.

Locally produced food has other benefits as well. It is fresher, riper and better-tasting, It is seasonal and thus provides essential variety in the diet. Buying local food is also more personal – you get to know the people who sell and produce your food. It also cuts down on air miles, which spew pollution into the air, which – apart from propelling us towards unrestrained global warming – eventually finds its way back into the food chain.

Eat organic
The increased demand for organic food has been the result of

many shifts in consumer consciousness. Food scares with regard to BSE and food-borne diseases have affected consumer confidence in conventional farming. Greater awareness of environmental issues has made many people make the ethical choice of eating organic foods. And the increasing use of alternative therapies that rely on organically grown foods has helped to renew interest in the quality of the food we eat.

Organic food contains, on average, higher levels of vitamin C and essential minerals such as calcium, magnesium, iron and chromium. Organic fruit and vegetables have higher levels (between 10 and 50 per cent) of secondary nutrients.[26] These include antioxidants that help to mop up the harmful free-radicals implicated in cancer. In a survey of organic vegetable soups, researchers found that they contained almost six times as much salicylic acid as non-organic vegetable soups. The acid helps to combat hardening of the arteries and bowel cancer, and is responsible for the anti-inflammatory action of aspirin. It is naturally used in plants as a defence against disease.

Eat the best quality you can afford

Avoid junk foods (such as biscuits, sweets and carbonated drinks), which are not only chock-full of artificial colouring and other additives, but are of little nutritional value – high in calories, sugar, fats and/or sodium. This is especially good advice for children, who are the main consumers of junk foods and are at increased risk if there are any health problems with additives. In addition, while freezing foods can be convenient, freezing also destroys vital nutrients, and there is even some indication that refrigeration has a similar effect.

Eat freshly prepared food

Consider removing the microwave from your kitchen. If you only use it to heat coffee, cook potatoes or pre-packaged meals, you probably don't need it. Getting rid of your microwave will also vastly improve the quality of the food you eat, since food that has been microwaved contains fewer nutrients. In addition, proteins, such as those found in meats, are significantly altered during the microwave process. Eating food directly from the microwave may also mean ingesting food that is still giving off radiation; this is why users are advised to let food 'sit' for a few minutes afterwards – to let all this radiation disperse.

Eat natural
If it comes in a box, tub, tray or jar – or if it is a colour that you don't normally see in nature – think twice before putting it in your mouth.

Eat variety
This may limit your exposure to any one additive – safer in the event that it turns out to have long-term health risks.

Eat seasonally
This is less expensive, provides greater variety in your diet and will reduce your exposure to antifungal and antibacterial chemicals that are commonly used to extend the shelf life of products grown out of season or shipped halfway across the globe.

Eat slowly
If it's a choice between a burger bar or the local café or restaurant, ditch the burger bar. If it's a choice between wolfing down a sandwich at your desk or sitting on a park bench, go to the park. Wherever possible, try to sit down and enjoy your meal and teach your children how to do the same.

Eat what you like

Be guided by your tastes, and be aware that the more you change your eating habits, the more your tastes will start to return to normal. Cravings for salty, sugary, highly processed foods will disappear and, with them, the tendency to overeat foods that are not good for your health.

These principles are the ABCs of good health and successful weight management. But, as the following chapter suggests, there is a wide and varied menu of supportive factors that can help you maintain a healthy weight and a healthy lifestyle.

CHAPTER 9

A menu for permanent weight loss

The premise of this book is that 21st-century life is having a marked and devastating effect on our health in general, and on our waistlines in particular. The modern world has brought many great things, and many new conveniences into our lives, and no one is suggesting that we all need to step back to the Stone Age in order to be healthy. Such a step would be impossible anyway, given how drastically we have altered ourselves and the world around us. Nevertheless, avoiding toxic exposure is arguably the single most important step to regaining your health.

When faced with the challenge of 'changing your lifestyle', most people don't know where to begin. It feels like an overwhelming task, and yet every effort you make will have a positive impact.

The pages that follow comprise a mix-and-match menu of things that anyone can do to help lessen the impact of the 21st century on their health. Many of these options have been proven to help minimize the effects of toxic exposure, either by reducing your exposure to them or by strengthening your body's ability to cope with them. Incorporate as many of these activities as you can, as often as you can, into your regular routine in order to improve your overall health and bolster your body's defences against a toxic world.

Avoid whatever toxins you can

You may not be able to control the environment outside your home, but you can control the environment inside your home. There are many sources of indoor pollution. Today, as we have seen, we ingest dozens of harmful chemicals when we eat conventionally grown produce: fertilizers, herbicides, pesticides and fungicides all combine to make so-called 'fresh' food a significant source of poisons. When we eat conventionally reared meats we are ingesting growth hormones and the myriad of 'just-in-case' medications given to conventionally farmed animals, in addition to the pesticides, herbicides, fertilizers and fungicides contained in their feed. As the BSE or 'mad-cow' saga has shown, we are sometimes also ingesting deadly micro-organisms.

Brightly coloured plastics in our homes may look modern and clean, but they continually give off toxic formaldehyde gas, which is implicated in respiratory problems and has been shown to be carcinogenic. Formaldehyde also comes from soft furnishings, vinyl wallpapers, insulation, varnishes, new carpets, upholstery and new mattresses.

Ever had a good whiff of a new book or newspaper? If so, you were inhaling toxic gases from the paper-processing and the ink. Thirsty? Tap water has become a significant source of many different toxins, including pesticides, hormones, hazardous waste and heavy metals, as well as water-borne parasites. If you live in an area where the water is fluoridated, your water contains a chemical that is more toxic than arsenic and only slightly less toxic than lead.

Given all this, you may wonder how we manage to stay healthy at all. The reality is that we don't. Even though we are now living longer than ever, we are strikingly unhealthy. Chronic diseases are on the rise, and obesity is just one piece of the puzzle of modern illness. Respiratory problems such as asthma and bronchitis have doubled in recent years, with the young being most affected. Vague disorders such as sinusitis and allergic rhinitis are becoming major problems, especially in inner-city areas. Heart disease, diabetes and thyroid problems are on the rise, too. Infertility (both male and female) is becoming more common, as are other hormonally linked disorders. Cancer continues to be a persistent disease across all cultures, age groups and genders, with no medical solution in sight.

The best way to minimize your exposure to environmental toxins is to consciously practise avoidance. This may mean identifying allergies and avoiding those things that trigger them. It may mean not inhaling nicotine, or overindulging in caffeine and alcohol. It may include avoiding toxic chemicals like fluoride and the volatile organic compounds found in most cleaning products, toiletries and perfumes. It may mean buying organic products, using natural wood in preference to plastic, using natural pest repellents in the home and garden, and seeking out paints and other types of home decoration that are low in toxins. You have more control over this than you probably realize, and doing whatever you can to lower your exposure to toxins will have a greatly beneficial effect on your health in both the short and the long term.

We are both passive and direct recipients of pollution, and none of us can avoid all poisons in the environment. But you do have more power than you think and you can, to a very large and influential extent, pick your poisons.

One way to do this is to be aware of what your particular weak spots are. These may be genetic weak spots, or ones developed in your own lifetime. For instance, if you have a family history of cancer, it makes sense to avoid carcinogenic chemicals and metals as far as possible. If your family has a history of neurological disorders (such as multiple sclerosis) or autoimmune diseases (such as arthritis), you should be on the look-out for neurotoxic and immunotoxic chemicals. If you suffer from menstrual problems, chemicals that disrupt your hormonal symptoms may play a part. If weight is your problem, then learning to avoid those chemicals that trigger weight gain is essential. Get to know what these chemicals are and make the effort to keep them out of your home, out of your diet and out of your life.

Chemicals in the carpet

The carpeting in your home is one of the major sources of neurotoxic VOCs such as 4-phenylcyclohexene, tetrachloroethylene, benzene, xylene, toluene, styrene and methylbenzenes. It is also a reservoir for pesticides, tobacco smoke and heavy metals.[1]

To find out just how prevalent these chemicals were in carpets, one laboratory in the US tested more than 400 carpet samples of varying age. They found these chemicals present in more than 90 per cent of samples tested.[2] Even samples 20 years old or more were still giving off neurotoxic and potentially fatal VOCs.

However, it's not just VOCs that lurk underfoot. Carpeting and house dust also harbour pesticides. In 1993 the Environmental Protection Agency (EPA)-sponsored Non-Occupational Pesticide Exposure Study (NOPES) was published.[3]

This study also confirmed that indoor air was more toxic than outdoor air, but instead of looking for VOCs, the NOPES study looked at pesticide levels. The researchers noted that, corresponding with the seasonal patterns of pesticide use, concentrations of pesticides in indoor air were highest in summer and lowest in winter. The most commonly detected pesticides were heptachlor, chlorpyrifos, aldrin, dieldrin, chlordane, atrazine, DDT, ortho-phenylphenol, propoxur, diazinon and carbaryl.

Most recently a report from the University of Exeter in the UK found that new carpets contain significant levels of the hormone-disrupting brominated flame-retardant BDE-209, as well as the pesticides permethrin (which was implicated in the debilitating symptoms suffered by Gulf War veterans) and tributyltin (an immune-system and reproductive toxin), as well as formaldehyde.[4]

Those most at risk from the pesticides in carpets are toddlers and infants, who spend much of their time in contact with the carpet, and who tend to put into their mouths things that have lain on the carpet. According to the NOPES study, this route of exposure provides infants and toddlers with nearly all non-dietary exposure to the neurotoxic, immunotoxic and endocrine-disturbing pesticides DDT, aldrin, atrazine and carbaryl.

Learn to breathe

Breathing properly can help clear the lungs and bloodstream of toxins. It is also relaxing and so lowers levels of stress hormones and encourages the immune system to work more efficiently. Getting more oxygen into the lungs is reputed to have the knock-on effect of improving the function of your eliminatory organs, such as the liver and kidneys, as well as your digestive tract. Oxygen-rich blood also feeds the nervous system, in particular the brain, which requires three times more oxygen to function than other organs in the body.

Unfortunately, most of us breathe in a shallow, inefficient way that reduces oxygen consumption and denies you the available benefits of breathing. When the breath is shallow, we are not taking in sufficient oxygen and are not eliminating sufficient carbon dioxide. As a result, our bodies become oxygen-starved, allowing toxins to build up. In addition, shallow breathing does not exercise the lungs sufficiently, and thus reduces their ability to function optimally, creating a vicious circle of lost vitality.

There are several reasons for the inefficient way that most of us breathe. These include:

• Fast-paced lifestyle. Where the body goes, the breath will follow. When our bodies and minds are in a rush, our breathing will also be rushed.

• Stress. When we are under stress, our fight-or-flight responses cause our breathing to become shallower.

• Emotions, such as depression, anxiety and fear, can affect the rate of breathing, causing it to be fast and shallow.

• Modern technology and automation reduce our need for physical activity. Without physical activity, there is little need to breathe deeply.

• Too much time spent indoors. We work and spend most of our leisure time indoors and this increases our exposure to pollution. In addition, there is a belief that when the body is in a polluted environment, it instinctively inhales less air – taking in just enough to tick over – to protect itself from the pollution.

The benefits of breathing correctly are receiving more and more scientific interest. Yogic breathing, or pranayama, which is slow and rhythmic and focuses on the out-breath, has, for example, produced a wide range of benefits in recent studies. Practices that involve breathing through the nostrils have been found to both stimulate and relax the sympathetic nervous system.[5] This type of breathing has also been found to be invigorating[6] and able to increase oxygen consumption and boost metabolism.[7] Yogic practice can also help with blood-glucose control.[8] Similarly, studies into Qigong breathing exercises have shown that these promote up to 20 per cent better oxygen consumption.[9]

To get the best out of deep breathing, try not to do it somewhere too polluted. Deep breathing on the high street or at the bus stop may not give your lungs the treat they need. Instead, take a walk in the park, get out into the country or go to the seaside. Better yet – and more convenient – make your home a toxin-free zone where you can practise deep-breathing exercises in peace and comfort. With practice, your breathing will become more efficient, naturally, wherever you are.

Try chelation

Chelation (pronounced *key-lay-shun*) therapy uses a variety of substances to remove toxic metals from the body. These substances bind to metals like lead, cadmium and arsenic, as well as other toxic substances, and help remove them from the body. Chelation therapy is extensively documented in medical literature, and is recognized as a legitimate treatment for lead poisoning. It has also been used to reverse hardening of the arteries.

The body does have its own natural chelation processes – digestion, assimilation, transport of food nutrients, and the formation of enzymes and hormones – as well as its own detoxification channels. However, when the amount of metal in the body becomes too high for the body to deal with by itself, chelation may be necessary.

The most well-known chelator is EDTA (ethylenediaminetetraacetic acid), an amino acid that is generally administered via an intravenous solution. EDTA binds to calcium deposits in the arteries and is used in cases of atherosclerosis, where it has a more than 80 per cent success rate. It can also remove lead (but not mercury) from the body. Intravenous EDTA is less expensive and less invasive than surgery, and there is evidence to suggest that it can also be useful for aneurysms, Alzheimer's disease and senile dementia, arthritis, autoimmune disorders, cancer, cataracts, diabetes, emphysema, gallstones, hypertension, kidney stones, Lou Gehrig's disease, osteoporosis, Parkinson's disease, scleroderma (a disease of the skin and connective tissue), strokes, varicose veins, venomous snake bites and other conditions involving an interruption in blood flow and diminished oxygen delivery.[10]

Intravenous EDTA is probably best reserved for those whose bodies are very polluted and who need urgent detoxification. Although non-toxic, EDTA can produce side-effects in some people. These include burning, redness and swelling at the injection site, fever, hypotension (low blood pressure), joint pain, skin outbreaks or rashes, upset stomach and, rarely, irritation of the kidneys and liver.[11] People who are debilitated, emaciated, have weak or diseased kidneys or advanced cardiovascular disease (end stage) are probably not good candidates for intravenous chelation, as a sudden, massive infusion of EDTA may put too much stress on the kidneys, liver and detoxification pathways in these individuals. However, there are some therapists who dispute this and say that professionally administered chelation poses little threat.

Stronger metal chelators, such as DMPS (2,3-dimercapto-1-propanesulphonic acid) or DMSA (dimercaptosuccinic acid), should only be used under a doctor's supervision and are even outlawed in some places.

Oral chelation using nutritional food supplements containing chelating agents (like EDTA, but also numerous natural chelators, such as vitamins, minerals, amino acids, antioxidants, phytonutrients and herbs) can also be effective, but will be a slower process. This is because only 4–18 per cent of an oral EDTA dose is absorbed (compared with 100 per cent of an intravenous dose).[12] Nevertheless, some oral chelation formulas have the ability to bond chemically with, and bring about the elimination of, mercury and other metals from the body. The addition of vitamins, minerals, enzymes and antioxidants may make oral chelation a less harmful process and more supportive of the body. While taking chelators, you should do all you can to support the body and avoid unnecessary sources of toxins.

Use (natural) functional foods

There are many so-called 'functional foods' on the market that claim to keep us healthy. Most contain what are known as pseudo-pharmaceuticals – synthetic substances that blur the lines between drugs and foods, enabling manufacturers to make extraordinary health claims (such as that a product lowers cholesterol). If at all possible, avoid these in favour of natural foods that have proven long-term benefits.

Consider these simple kitchen-cupboard solutions to combat

everyday toxins:

• Pectin, found in apple and pear seeds, can protect your body from damage by toxic metals. It works by blocking the absorption of toxins, while aiding detoxification. Try making apples or pears that have been stewed with their seeds a regular feature of your diet.

• Garlic and onions contain powerful antioxidants that aid the body's natural day-to-day efforts to detox. Use them liberally in cooking. Other sulphur-rich foods (such as broccoli) and bile-stimulants (such as lemon) and bitter greens also assist in detoxi-fication.

• Peas, beans and lentils contain unique antioxidants, and are high in fibre, which can bind to toxins and aid their excretion from the body. Pulses are a good alternative source of protein, so why not substitute a couple of meat meals each week with one based on (organic) pulses.

• A high-fibre diet is useful in general for trapping toxins and assisting in the elimination of heavy metals. Fibre helps to reduce intestinal permeability, sometimes known as 'leaky gut' – a condition that can lead to allergies and toxic build-up in the bloodstream. It also prevents deactivated oestrogens from being reactivated and reabsorbed. Consider adding to your diet water-soluble, mucilaginous (moist and sticky) fibres such as psyllium seeds and flax seeds. These can be ground up and added to cereals, soups and baked foods.

• Bananas have antioxidant qualities.

• Eggs protect against lead and mercury contamination.

• All leafy, dark green vegetables, but especially cruciferous vegetables (those belonging to the cabbage family), can inhibit the carcinogenic effects of chemicals. Try to include plenty of kale, spinach, broccoli and Brussels sprouts in your diet. Other green foods such as chlorophyll are also natural chelators, able to draw heavy metals out of the system.[13] Herbs like coriander (cilantro) are another sound choice. A good way to get your greens is to buy a juicer and use it to make vegetable juices – they are not as sweet as fruit juices, but they pack more punch in the detox stakes.

• Seaweeds and alginates may also bind to heavy metals. There is evidence, for instance, that chlorella can draw persistent chemicals such as PCBs out of the system.[14] Similarly, research stretching back several decades shows that Arctic seaweeds are an aid to detoxification.[15] These can be taken as supplements or added to your diet.

• Black tea is also thought to provide some protection from heavy-metal toxicity – but the evidence so far comes only from animals. Similar results are likely to occur with green tea.

Get juicing

Fruit juices are tasty, but – even freshly squeezed ones – are full of sugar; when it comes to detoxing, they cannot compare with the powerful effect of vegetable juices. Having said that, you need to be choosy about which vegetables you select. Veggie juices made from carrots and beetroot taste good, but are as full of sugar as most fruit juices.

Mild detox drinks can be made from greens such as celery, fennel (anise) and cucumber. This is a good way to introduce yourself to the taste and effects of vegetable juices if you've never had them before.

However, it is the dark green, leafy (though sometimes less palatable) vegetable juices that will benefit you most. This is partly because of their chlorophyll content and partly because of their high antioxidant content. Once you get used to the milder juices, you can introduce more powerful mixtures made from lettuces such as red leaf, green leaf, romaine and endive, as well as other greens, like escarole, spinach, cabbage, Chinese cabbage and pak choi (bok choy).

Adding herbs like parsley and coriander (cilantro) to the juices will impart flavour to them, as well as furthering their detox benefits. Start with small amounts and monitor your body's responses.

Other types of greens that you can use (sparingly, because they are very bitter) include kale, collard greens, dandelion greens and mustard greens. Make sure that you wash all your greens thoroughly before juicing and, where possible, buy organic for even greater benefit.

Keep your carbohydrates complex

Fear of fat has led to widespread acceptance of the carbohydrate as the keep-fit generation's official 'best' food. As dietary fat consumption has dropped, so carbohydrate consumption has skyrocketed. But instead of becoming leaner, body weights have continued to rise. Part of the problem is hidden carbohydrates. Cereals and pulses are sources of carbohydrates, but so are vegetables, fruit, sugar, nuts, seeds, fruit juices and milk.

Carbohydrates are known as energy foods because, when metabolized, they supply glucose, a sugar that circulates in our blood, providing energy where the body needs it. Our muscles, and especially our brains, need glucose in order to function.

But just because carbohydrates are low in fat doesn't mean they are automatically good for keeping thin. Although they contain fewer calories than fat, they are also more easily stored as fat if they are consumed in excess. The body produces insulin in response to the rise in blood sugar that carbohydrates produce. Insulin removes excess glucose and stores it, first as glycogen and then as fat. If we overconsume carbohydrates, especially high levels of refined-grain products such as bread, more insulin is produced and more fat is stored. High insulin levels promote fat storage and block the release of fat-burning glucagon. Even though carbohydrates are in themselves fat-free, they can eventually be stored as fat and prevent your body from burning fat.

Researchers at Harvard School of Public Health found that replacing fats with a high-carbohydrate diet lowered both 'bad' LDL (low-density lipoprotein) and 'good' HDL (high-density lipoprotein) cholesterol and reduced vitamin E and essential fatty acids. The researchers claimed that there is no proof that a low-fat, high-carbohydrate diet reduces the risk of cancer or helps maintain body weight.[16] Interestingly, a study published years ago in *The Lancet* actually showed that people on a 2,600-calorie-per-day diet with a low intake of carbohydrates would lose weight, despite the higher fat content of the diet.[17]

Overconsuming carbohydrates doesn't just affect your weight. Consider that:

• Refined carbohydrates are not much more than simple sugars. They have an often-dramatic effect on insulin levels and can lead to depression and anxiety.

• These sugars also wreak havoc on the immune system.

• Carbohydrates in the form of wheat are linked with allergies. They have also been linked with cancer, osteoporosis, hypoglycaemia, adrenal exhaustion and parasitic and yeast infections.

• Overconsumption of carbohydrates is also associated with a greater number of food cravings – often resulting in binge-eating.

Nevertheless, carbohydrates are essential to life. And not all carbohydrates have the same effect on insulin secretion. Complex carbohydrates such as those found in whole grains take longer to digest and are less likely to be stored as fats. The slower speed at which they are broken down by digestion means that you maintain a much more constant blood-sugar level.

Ditch the TV

We don't make our own entertainment any more. Instead we have it sent to us down cables and wires. Television, watched selectively, can be a wonderful source of entertainment and a window on the world. But these days most of us just turn it on as background noise for hours at a time, happy to watch 24-hour news programmes that repeat the same stories over and over again and channels that repeatedly broadcast sitcom and soap-opera reruns.

Too much TV has been linked to obesity, in adults and especially in children.[18] Evidence suggests that a child's weight increases with the number of hours he or she spends watching television each day.[19]

Experts label television viewing as the number-one leisuretime activity of most school-age children. The problem stems from the fact that watching television is a sedentary activity – but it's much more than that. Children are watching TV, often while eating high-calorie/high-fat snack foods, and watching commercials for fast food, all of which may encourage even more eating.

It is worth remembering, too, that TV does more than promote lack of exercise and snacking. By presenting viewers with an unreal world of perfection and hard-to-achieve aspirations (about how we should look and how we should interact with each other), television can sap a person's motivation to participate in the real world. As often as possible, get out into that real world – with all its problems and faults, it is still much more interesting and entertaining than the virtual one.

Get tested

There are a number of tests that you can undergo to check the levels of metals and other poisons in your body. Hair analysis –

which usually involves taking a small sample of recent hair growth from the nape of the neck – is a common way of testing for the presence of heavy metals. A lab analysis can give you fairly accurate information on the presence of calcium, magnesium, sodium, potassium, iron, copper, manganese, zinc, chromium and selenium, but also on potentially more damaging metals, such as lead, mercury, cadmium and arsenic.

Some practitioners also offer blood- and urine-testing, although these have been shown to be less effective in the detection of minerals and, especially, toxic-metal exposure. This is because blood shows what is being transported in the body, while urine shows what is being eliminated. Stool-testing, however, can be useful for diagnosing the presence of parasites in the gut.

To test for allergies, practitioners use either a skin-prick test or blood analysis such as the RAST (radioallergosorbent test) or the ELISA (enzyme-linked immunosorbent assay). These last two are based on the idea that, when the body registers an allergen in its midst, it produces a variety of immunoglobulin antibodies. Both tests look for the presence of antibodies, although there is continuing debate about how useful either (or, indeed, any) of the current test methods is, since different tests performed by different laboratories on the same samples of blood can produce sometimes wildly different results. Many pharmacies now sell over-the-counter tests, but these are unlikely to be very accurate. For a better chance of success you need to visit an allergy specialist who has access to a reliable laboratory.

In the UK few of these tests are offered on the National Health Service. You will need to seek out a private practitioner to have them performed, just as you will in the US, unless you are covered by medical insurance.

Take exercise seriously

Whether exercise promotes serious weight loss is still in dispute. But the fact is that our bodies are designed to be used. When we don't use them to their optimal extent, muscles deteriorate, metabolism becomes sluggish and breathing becomes shallow. For all these reasons it is desirable to develop good, sensible habits of exercise – whether these are aerobic routines, an active lifestyle or weight-training – that you can easily incorporate into your life for the rest of your life.

Over the years many studies have documented the positive benefits of regular exercise. For instance, physically active individuals have:

• Lower rates of heart disease[20]
• Less depression and anxiety[21]
• Better blood-pressure control[22]
• Better glucose control[23]
• Reduced joint swelling in those with arthritis[24]
• Lower risk of colon cancer[25] and diverticular disease,[26] as well as other cancers
• Fewer gallstones[27]
• Reduced risk of bone fracture[28]
• Better sleep quality[29]
• Better mental health[30]
• Greater enthusiasm for life[31]
• Maintenance of their ideal weight[32]
• Longer lifespan (on average seven years longer).[33]

Studies also show that regular aerobic exercise can help to detoxify the body.[34] For instance, in a study of firemen exposed to toxic PCBs, a two- to three-week detox programme that involved diet, daily saunas and 30–60 minutes of exercise twice weekly helped to remove these highly toxic substances from their bodies more quickly.[35]

Research has also found that the less muscle you have, the harder it is to lose weight, because muscle is metabolically active, but body fat is inactive. Therefore, when women diet but don't exercise, 25 per cent of any weight lost is made up of water, muscle, bone and other lean tissue. Muscle mass uses up more calories than fat: up to 30–50 calories a day, compared with only two calories a day for fat.

Exercise does not have to be onerous. Walking around a shopping mall is just as healthy as walking around the block.[36] Indeed, walking is really an ideal and natural form of exercise in which anyone can routinely participate.[37] It also provides direct contact with the elements and nature, which can be calming and refreshing to the senses. Walking is a load-bearing exercise that tones muscles, improves fitness, circulation, appetite and breathing.

Other evidence suggests that washing and waxing the car and other household activities, when undertaken regularly, can extend your life. All it takes is 30 minutes of moderate activity (essentially anything that produces a moderate sweat) each day.[38]

Similarly, gentle regimes such as yoga and Qigong have demonstrated benefits. In studies, Qigong practitioners have shown increased immunity response,[39] improved mental concentration and greater calm.

Don't overdo it

It is possible to take exercise too seriously. Overtraining can lead to physical injuries, but it can also encourage oxidative stress. The more energetic and long-lasting your exercise, the more oxygen you take into your body. During intense exercise, we can take in up to 20 times the normal volume of oxygen. This is generally considered a good thing, but more oxygen also means increased demands on the body as it struggles to metabolize all this extra oxygen. The result is a well-known, but little-publicized, adverse effect of intensive training – oxidative stress and the production of muscle- and organ-damaging free-radicals.

Overtraining can also lead to imbalances in the stress hormone cortisol (see Chapter 7). Within the normal range, cortisol can have protective effects on the body. But too much or too little can have important effects on health. When levels are high, strength can start to decrease;[40] when levels are low, there is a marked inability to deal with other stressors.[41] Cortisol metabolism is also a source of free-radicals that are implicated in premature ageing and degenerative diseases.

A huge amount of data exists on the benefits of being physically active. As we have seen, a physically active person has a life expectancy that is on average seven years longer.[42] He or she will be prone to less depression and anxiety, and will experience better mental efficiency,[43] higher self-esteem,[44] more restful sleep,[45] more relaxation, spontaneity, enthusiasm and better self-acceptance in both adults[46] and children.[47]

But is there one definitive type of exercise that is of universal benefit? It may be, as in everything else, that exercise needs to be tailored to individual requirements. For the man or woman whose heart health is an issue, 20 minutes of aerobic exercise three times a week may work as a preventative. For the woman who is at risk of osteoporosis, weight-bearing exercises that do not put excessive strain on the joints are a better choice.

Don't worry too much about which activities burn more calories. There are always swings and roundabouts. Weight-bearing activities that work against gravity – aerobic activities such as walking, running, cross-country skiing, dancing, skating and stair-climbing – use proportionately more calories at a given level of effort than swimming, cycling or water aerobics. The more muscle groups involved in your activities, the more calories you are likely to burn. That is why working out against gravity uses more calories than non-weight-bearing activities. On the other hand, because activities like swimming put less stress on weight-bearing joints, many people can do them for longer periods, making up for the lower caloric burn.

Some people compensate for the calories burned by eating more or doing less. If you exhaust yourself by overexercising, you may do less routine activity for the rest of the day, reducing the caloric benefit of your workout, so don't overdo it (see also box on pages 201–202) – and remember that you don't need to go at it hard to reap the benefits.

In fact, there may even be a metabolic advantage to periods of rest in between bouts of exercise. According to a 2007 Japanese study, allowing time for a rest period during your workout burns more fat than exercising for one continuous session of activity.[48] The unprecedented study compared the workout sessions of seven healthy men with an average age of 25. Their respiratory gas and heart rates were monitored, and blood samples taken, while they performed the following scenarios:

• A 60-minute workout on a cycling machine, followed by a 60-minute rest period (single)

• Two 30-minute workouts on a cycling machine with a 20-minute rest in between, and a 60-minute recovery period at the end (repeated)

• A 60-minute rest period (for control purposes).

It was found that the participants had a greater amount of fat breakdown, or lipolysis, during the repeated session than during the single session.

Meanwhile, the repeated trial caused a greater increase in free fatty acids and glycerol, which are released when stored fat is burned, than did the single trial. Also during the repeated session, levels of the hormone epinephrine increased and levels of insulin decreased far more than during the single session – a combination that may have further contributed to fat breakdown.

Drink water

But drink it intelligently. Most of us have grown up with the idea that we should drink eight 250 ml (8 fl oz) glasses (approximately 1.8 litres/3 pints) of water a day in order to stay healthy. Certainly water is an essential and often-overlooked nutrient,[49] but outside of the field of sports medicine it is almost impossible to find good evidence to support the eight-glasses-a-day theory. Few of us are actually training for the triathlon (endurance sports are probably the only situation where overconsumption of water, such as drinking up to 1 litre/1¾ pints prior to extreme exertion, may be justified) and information about how much fluid sedentary to moderately active individuals need is less clear-cut.[50]

In the same way that adequate nutrition has little to do with how many vitamin pills you take, so adequate hydration is not just a matter of drinking lots of water. It is a question of checks and balances. How much you need depends on various factors, such as your level of activity, what kind of foods you regularly consume and even the climate in which you live.

It is estimated that, every day, the body loses approximately 1.5 litres/2½ pints of water through sweating, breathing and urinating. This water must be replaced. The good news is that your daily fluid supply doesn't all have to come from a bottle or a glass. Fruit and vegetables supply water in a form that is easily used by the body, while providing a high percentage of vitamins and minerals as a bonus.

In addition, we release about 300 ml (½ pint) of water into our systems every day when we burn glycogen for energy. When the body digests carbohydrates, they are broken down into glucose – to meet immediate energy needs – and glycogen. Glycogen is stored in the muscles and liver for future use. Each molecule of glycogen holds on to nine molecules of water, which are released during the course of your day and at times when you need it most, such as during intense exercise.

Increasing your fluid intake too dramatically can put unnecessary stress on your kidneys and digestive system. So, if you want to increase your daily intake, try adding one 300 ml (½ pint) glass of water every other day until you are drinking as much as you need.

You may also wish to consider the following:

• If you find that drinking water makes you feel too full, you may be gulping down large quantities of air each time you swallow. To remedy this, try drinking through a straw.

• The idea that you can dilute your digestive juices by drinking water with a meal is a myth. Every day, the body makes about 10 litres (17 pints) of digestive juices. A glass of water with your food won't even make a dent in this.

• Before engaging in vigorous exercise, try drinking at least 300 ml (½ pint) of water beforehand. Keep a water bottle with you, and drink 125–250 ml (4–8 fl oz) every 15 minutes or so to maintain your body temperature and avoid dehydration.

• Lots of people limit the amount of fluids they drink each day because they want to limit the number of times they go to the toilet. But going to the toilet every two to four hours is a sign of good health. After a few weeks your bladder will adapt, you will go to the toilet less frequently and, when you do, you will void larger amounts of pale urine.

• While is it sensible to be guided by your appetite where food is concerned, being guided by your thirst is not a good idea. Regardless of your level of activity, by the time you feel thirsty, you are already partially dehydrated. To avoid this, sip water throughout the day and get into the habit of drinking this in preference to potentially drying liquids such as coffee, tea and carbonated drinks. This and increasing your intake of 'watery' foods (see below) will ensure that your body is getting what it needs – without having to carry around heavy designer bottles of water.

Water content of food

A single serving of any of the items below can count towards your total daily fluid intake:

Food	Water (%)
Lettuce	95.5
Kale	91.2
Carrots	91.2
Milk	87.5
Porridge	86.5
Apples	84.4
Grapes	81.6
Potatoes, baked in their skins	75.1
Brown rice, cooked	70.3
Beans such as kidney beans or lentils, cooked	70.0
Fish or chicken, grilled	64.0

Sports drinks help to replace lost electrolytes (salts) and provide useful levels of sodium, potassium and quick energy in the form of glucose. However, unless you are involved in regular and very heavy workouts, you are unlikely to need to replace electrolytes. For moderately active people, sports drinks probably only offer more calories and less benefit. A regular, wholesome diet will provide the average person with all the electrolytes they need, as well as essential nutrients.

Those who are taking multivitamin/mineral supplements should make sure they are adequately hydrated, as should those who engage in regular sweaty workouts. Do sip water when exercising, even if you don't feel thirsty. During a hard workout, by the time you feel thirsty you may already be dehydrated.

You also need extra water in warmer weather, when you are running a fever and when you have diarrhoea.

What type of water is best?

The quality of the water we drink is almost as important as the quantity. As a general recommendation, for the best-quality water, consider installing a reverse-osmosis filter at your own tap (but be careful, because some of these use plastic filters, which can leech chemicals into your drinking water). Beyond that, there are benefits and limitations to every type of water that you choose to drink. No home-filter process is infallible. Distilled water is pure, but may be lacking in certain minerals. Jug filters have to do what they claim on the label; this means that they do filter out a substantial amount of contaminants such as chlorine and heavy metals,[51] but with use they can also become reservoirs for bacteria.[52]

While some local water authorities seem to be able to produce clean drinkable water, others cannot, and contamination with heavy metals, bacteria and parasites such as *Cryptosporidium* is becoming an increasing concern. Nevertheless, if you have confidence in your local water supply, tap water does have its benefits – the main one being that it is almost always available. In addition, if you get into the habit of drinking only bottled water, you can easily reach a point where you believe that when the bottle is empty, you've run out of water.

Bottled waters can be high in minerals, and chemicals from the plastic bottle may leech into the water during storage. There is little evidence that bottled waters are substantially healthier for you to drink than tap water, though they are (sometimes) convenient.[53]

And finally ... embrace life

None of the things suggested in this chapter are possible unless you actually enjoy living. Indeed, self-esteem, social ties and life satisfaction are amongst those things that most influence the way we take care of ourselves over the long haul.[54] Similarly, a sense of productivity and worth, and faith in a god or higher power, have also been shown to be influential.[55]

Curiosity and taking an interest in the world around you may also have an important role to play,[56] as does your personality. But, contrary to common perceptions, this does not necessarily mean that the most cheerful and optimistic personalities survive the longest. In one study, cheerfulness (defined as optimism and a sense of humour) was linked to early death, while conscientiousness (attention to details) was related to longevity.[57] Other research along similar lines has shown that stability of personality and a sense of routine may be the most important factors.[58]

These ideas are underscored by the findings from a retrospective study in which the factors influencing 17 long-surviving American Civil War nurses in the late 19th century, including Louisa May Alcott, Dorothea Dix and Clara Barton, were explored. While social and marital status, altruism and religion were all important, more than any other tangible factor the presence of a pioneering spirit seemed to lie at the root of their longevity.[59]

Clearly, when you enjoy life, when you have people around you whom you care about and who care about you, when your work is interesting and challenging and your mind is free to follow its own thoughts, you become interested in living. You will then have good reason to do all you can to protect yourself and your loved ones from an increasingly toxic environment.

Notes

Introduction: A 21st-century problem

1 Hedley, A.A. et al., 'Prevalence of overweight and obesity among US children, adolescents, and adults 1999–2002', *Journal of the American Medical Association*, 2004, vol. 291: 2847–50

2 World Health Organization, *The World Health Report: Reducing Risks, Promoting Healthy Life*, WHO, 2002

3 World Health Organization, *Obesity: Preventing and Managing the Global Epidemic. Report of WHO Consultation on Obesity*, WHO, 1998

4 Popkin, Prof. Barry, University of North Carolina, addressing the International Association of Agricultural Economists, Brisbane, Australia, August 2006; BBC News report online at: *http://news.bbc.co.uk/1/hi/health/4793455.stm*

5 Tanaka, K., Nakanishi, T., 'Obesity as a risk factor for various diseases: Necessity of lifestyle changes for healthy aging', *Applied Human Science*, 1996, vol. 15 (4): 139–48

6 American Academy of Pediatrics, 'Prevention of pediatric overweight and obesity', *Pediatrics*, 2003, vol. 112 (2): 424–30; Mishra, V., 'Effect of obesity on asthma among adult Indian women', *International Journal of Obesity*, 2004, vol. 28: 1048–58; Saw, S.M., Rajan, U., 'The epidemiology of obesity: A review', *Annals of the Academy of Medicine, Singapore*, 1997, vol. 26 (4): 489–93

7 Shannon, M., 'An empathetic look at overweight', *CCL Family Foundations*, 1993, vol. 20 (3): 3

8 Finkelstein, E.A. et al., 'National medical spending attributable to overweight and obesity: How much, and who's paying?', *Health Affairs*, 2003, vol. W3: 219–26

9 *Health Survey for England 2004*, National Centre for Social Research, 2005

10 Prentice, A.M., Jebb, S.A., 'Obesity in Britain: Gluttony or sloth?', *British Medical Journal*, 1995, vol. 311: 437–39

11 Cannon, G., 'Dieting. Makes you fat?', *British Journal of Nutrition*, 2005, vol. 93: 569–70

12 Sweeney, M.E. et al., 'Severe vs moderate energy restriction with and without exercise in the treatment of obesity: Efficiency of weight loss', *American Journal of Clinical Nutrition*, 1993, vol. 57: 127–34

13 Calles-Escandón, J., Horton, E.S., 'The thermogenic role of exercise in the treatment of morbid obesity: A critical evaluation', *American Journal of Clinical Nutrition*, 1992, vol. 55: 533S–7S

14 Dr Foster Intelligence, 'Legacy of ex-industrial towns revealed in latest survey of obesity', 31 August 2006; online news release available at: *http://www.drfosterintelligence.co.uk/newsPublications/article.asp?articleid=18&from=archive*

15 Hawkes, N., 'Fat map pinpoints the streets with a weight problem', *The Times*, 1 September 2006

16 *F as in Fat 2006: How Obesity Policies are Failing in America*, Trust for America's Health, 2006

17 Keith, S.W. et al., 'Putative contributors to the secular increase in obesity: Exploring the roads less travelled', *International Journal of Obesity*, 2006, advance online publication, 27 June 2006, doi:10.1038/sj.ijo.0803326

Chapter 1: How dieting fails us

1 Mann, T. et al., 'Medicare's search for effective obesity treatments: Diets are not the answer', *American Psychologist*, April 2007, vol. 62(3): 220–33

2 Lissner, L. et coll., 'Variability of body weight and health outcomes in the Framingham population', *New England Journal*

of Medicine, 1991, vol. 324: 1839–44

3 Rexrode, K. et al., 'A prospective study of body mass index, weight change, and risk of stroke in women', *Journal of the American Medical Association*, 21 May 1997, vol. 277(19): 1539–45; Willett, W.C., Manson, J.E., Stampfer, M.J., Colditz, G.A., Rosner, B., Speizer, F.E. et al., 'Weight, weight change and coronary heart disease in women', *Journal of the American Medical Association*, 1995, vol. 273: 461–65

4 Wannameethee, G., Shaper, A.G., 'Weight change in middle-aged British men: Implications for health', *European Journal of Clinical Nutrition*, 1990, vol. 44: 133–42; Higgins, 'Benefits and adverse effects of weight loss', *Annals of Internal Medicine*, 1993, vol. 119: 758–63

5 Losonczy, K.G. et al., 'Does weight loss from middle age to old age explain the inverse weight mortality relation in old age?', *American Journal of Epidemiology*, 1995, vol. 141(4): 312–21

6 Langlois, J.A. et al., 'Weight change between age 50 years and old age is associated with risk of hip fracture in white women aged 67 years and older', *Archives of Internal Medicine*, 1996, vol. 156: 989–94

7 Andres, R., Muller, D.C., Sorkin, J.D., 'Long-term effects of change in body weight on all-cause mortality. A review', *Annals of Internal Medicine*, 1993, vol. 119: 737–43

8 Toubro, S., Astrup, A., 'Randomised comparison of diets for maintaining obese subjects' weight after major weight loss: Ad lib, low fat, high carbohydrate diet v fixed energy intake', *British Medical Journal*, 1997, vol. 314 (7073): 29–34

9 Cannon, G., 'Dieting. Makes you fat?', *British Journal of Nutrition*, 2005, vol. 93: 569–70

10 Brownell, K.D. et al., 'The effects of repeated cycles of weight loss and regain in rats', *Physiology and Behavior*, 1986, vol. 38: 459–64

11 Steen, S.N. et al., 'Metabolic effects of repeated weight loss and regain in adolescent wrestlers', *Journal of the American Medical Association*, 1988, vol. 260: 47–50

12 Stice, E. et al., 'Naturalistic weight-reduction efforts prospectively predict growth in relative weight and onset of obesity among female adolescents', *Journal of Consulting and Clinical Psychology*, 1999, vol. 67: 967–74

13 Field, A.E. et al., 'Relation between dieting and weight change among preadolescents and adolescents', *Pediatrics*, 2003, vol. 112: 900–06

14 CNN Interactive, 'Survey: Many opt for high-protein, low-carb diets', 4 March 1999; online at: *www.cnn.com/HEALTH/9903/04/diet.survey/*

15 Moynihan, R. and Cassels, A., *Selling Sickness: How the World's Biggest Pharmaceutical Companies Are Turning Us All into Patients*, Allen & Unwin, 2005; Law, J., *Big Pharma*, Constable and Robinson, 2006

16 'The U.S. Weight Loss & Diet Control Market', Marketdata Enterprises, Inc., March 2005

17 'Diet Watchers 2003', *Datamonitor*, 12 November 2003

18 'The Clinical Guidelines on the Identification, Evaluation and Treatment of Overweight and Obesity in Adults: Evidence Report', National Heart, Lung and Blood Institute, National Institutes of Health, US Department of Health and Human Services, September 1998, NIH pub. no. 98-4083

19 Connolly, M.D. et al., 'Valvular heart disease associated with fenfluramine-phentermine', *New England Journal of Medicine*, 1997, vol. 337: 581–88; see also Abenhaim, M.D. et al., 'Appetite-suppressant drugs and the risk of primary pulmonary hypertension', *New England Journal of Medicine*, 1996, vol. 335: 609–16

20 Stein, R., 'CDC study overestimated deaths from obesity',

Washington Post, 24 November 2004, page A11

21 Flegal, K.M. et al., 'Excess deaths associated with underweight, overweight, and obesity', *Journal of the American Medical Association*, 2005, vol. 293: 1861–67

22 'Obesity and the facts – An analysis of data from the Health Survey for England 2003', Social Issues Research Centre, February 2005; online at: *www.sirc.org/obesity/obesityfacts.pdf*

23 Oliver, E., *Fat Politics – The Real Story Behind America's Obesity Epidemic*, Oxford University Press, 2005

24 Patton, G.C. et al, 'Onset of adolescent eating disorders: Population-based cohort study over 3 years', *British Medical Journal*, 1999, vol. 318: 765–68

25 Story, M. et al, 'Demographic and risk factors associated with chronic dieting in adolescents', *American Journal of Diseases of Children*, 1991, vol. 145: 994–98; Neumark-Sztainer, D., Butler, R., Palti, H., 'Dieting and binge eating: Which dieters are at risk?', *Journal of the American Dietetic Association*, 1995, vol. 95: 586–89

26 Polivy, J., 'Psychological consequences of food restriction', *Journal of the American Dietetic Association*, 1996, vol. 96: 589–92

27 Lifshitz, F. et al, 'Nutritional dwarfing in adolescents', *Seminars in Adolescent Medicine*, 1987, vol. 3: 255–66; Pugliese, M. et al, 'Fear of obesity. A cause of short stature and delayed puberty', *New England Journal of Medicine*, 1983, vol. 309: 513–18; Dietz, W.H. Jr, Hartung, R., 'Changes in height velocity of obese preadolescents during weight reduction', *American Journal of Diseases of Children*, 1985, vol. 139: 705-07

28 Selzer, R. et al, 'The association between secondary amenorrhea and common eating disordered weight control practices in an adolescent population', *Journal of Adolescent Health*, 1996, vol. 19: 56–61; Kriepe, R.E., Forbes, G.B.,

'Osteoporosis: A new morbidity for dieting female adolescence?', *Pediatrics*, 1990, vol. 86: 478–80; Johnson, J., Whitaker, A.H., 'Adolescent smoking, weight changes, and binge-purge behavior: Associations with secondary amenorrhea', *American Journal of Public Health*, 1992, vol. 82: 47–54; Kreipe, R.E., et al, 'Menstrual cycle abnormalities and subclinical eating disorders: A preliminary report', *Psychosomatic Medicine*, 1989, vol. 51: 81–86

29 Turner, J.M. et al,'Predictors of low bone density in young adolescent females with anorexia nervosa and other dieting disorders', *International Journal of Eating Disorders*, 2001, vol. 30: 245–51

30 'Dieting Can Slow Reaction Time, Food and Nutrition Research Briefs', USDA/ARS, April 1997; online: *www.ars.usda.gov/is/np/fnrb/fnrb497.htm*

31 Pond, C.M., *The Fats of Life*, Cambridge University Press, 1998

32 Pond, C.M., 'Long-term changes in adipose tissue in human disease', *Proceedings of the Nutrition Society*, 2001, vol. 60: 365–74

33 Angier, N., 'Fat on thighs and paunches is the fate of all mammals', *New York Times*, 30 October 1990

34 Freidman, J.M., 'The function of leptin in nutrition, weight and physiology', *Nutrition Reviews*, 2002, vol. 11 (supplement): 1–14; Halaas, J.L., Gajiwala, K.S., Maffei, M. et al., 'Weight reducing effects of the plasma protein encoded by the obese gene', *Science*, 1995, vol. 269: 543–46

35 Bouret, S.G. et al., 'Trophic action of leptin on hypothalamic neurons that regulate feeding', *Science*, 2004, vol. 304, 110–15; Pinto, S. et al., 'Rapid rewiring of arcuate nucleus feeding circuits by leptin', *Science*, 2004, vol. 304: 110–15; Elmquist, J.K., Flier, J.S., 'The fat-brain axis enters a new dimension', *Science*, 2004,

vol. 304: 110–15

36 Bates, S.H. et al., 'Roles for leptin receptor/STAT3-dependent and -independent signals in the regulation of glucose homeostasis', *Cell Metabolism*, March 2005, vol. 1: 169–78

37 Hoda, M.R. et al., 'Leptin acts as a mitogenic and antiapoptotic factor for colonic cancer cells', *British Journal of Surgery*, 2007, vol. 94: 346–54

Chapter 2: The bigger picture

1 'Diet, Nutrition and the Prevention of Chronic Diseases. Report of a joint WHO/FAO expert consultation', *Technical Report Series*, no. 916, World Health Organization, 2003; Bell, A.C. et al., 'The road to obesity or the path to prevention: Motorized transportation and obesity in China', *Obesity Research*, 2002, vol. 10 (4): 277–83; Popkin, B.M., 'The nutrition transition and its health implications in lower-income countries', *Public Health Nutrition*, 1998, vol. 1: 5–21; Popkin, B.M., 'Nutrition in transition: The changing global nutrition challenge', *Asia Pacific Journal of Clinical Nutrition*, 2001, vol. 10 (supplement): S13–S18; Popkin, B.M., 'The shift in stages of the nutritional transition in the developing world differs from past experiences', *Public Health Nutrition*, 2002, vol. 5(1A): 205–14; Popkin, B.M. et al., 'Trends in diet, nutritional status, and diet-related noncommunicable diseases in China and India: The economic costs of the nutrition transition', *Nutrition Reviews*, 2001, vol. 59 (12): 379–90; Drewnowski, A., Popkin, B.M., 'The nutrition transition: New trends in the global diet', *Nutrition Reviews*, 1997, vol. 55 (2): 31–43

2 Foley, M., 'Western ag policies blamed for obesity', *Forbes* magazine, 4 September 2006; online at *www.cbsnews.com/stories/2006/09/05/ap/health/mainD8JUCTMG0.shtml*; see also Popkin, B.M., 'The nutrition transition and obesity in the

developing world', *Journal of Nutrition*, 2001, vol. 131: 871S–73S

3 Hui, S., Chinese University of Hong Kong press release, 25 May 2007; online at: *www.cuhk.edu.hk/cpr/pressrelease/070525e.htm*

4 Agrawal, P., 'Role of lifestyle and diet in emerging obesity among Indian women and its impact upon their health status', Paper presented in the IUSSP XXV International Population Conference, Tours, France, 18–23 July 2005

5 Schlosser, E., *Fast Food Nation: The Dark Side of the American Meal*, Penguin Books, 2002

6 Reilly, J.J. et al., 'Physical activity to prevent obesity in young children: Cluster randomised controlled trial', *British Medical Journal*, 2006, vol. 333: 1041–45

7 Keller, C., 'Review: Dietary intervention plus exercise is no better than dietary intervention alone for inducing long term weight loss', *Evidence-Based Nursing*, 2006, vol. 9 (2): 46–7

8 La Forge, R., 'Exercise Determinants of Weight Loss: Key Considerations for Metabolic Syndrome and Diabetes Prevention Programs', *ACE Certified News*, August/September 2006

9 'Diet, Nutrition and the Prevention of Chronic Diseases. Report of a joint WHO/FAO expert consultation', *Technical Report Series*, no. 916, World Health Organization, 2003; 'The Asia-Pacific Perspective: Redefining Obesity and its Treatment. Report of the International Association for the Study of Obesity (IASO) and International Obesity Task Force (IOTF)', World Health Organization, 2000

10 Marsh, P., 'Poverty and obesity', Social Issues Research Centre, 15 March 2004; online at: *www.sirc.org/articles/poverty_and_obesity.shtml*

11 *Obesity among adults: By sex and NS-SeC, 2001, Social Trends 34*, Office of National Statistics, February 2004

12 Kinra, S. et al., 'Deprivation and childhood obesity: A cross sectional study of 20,973 children in Plymouth, United Kingdom', *Journal of Epidemiology and Community Health*, 2000, vol. 54: 456–60

13 'Health Survey for England: Cardiovascular Disease '98', Joint Health Surveys Unit on behalf of the Department of Health, The Stationery Office, 1999

14 'Health Survey for England: The Health of Minority Ethnic Groups '99', Joint Health Surveys Unit on behalf of the Department of Health, The Stationery Office, 2001

15 Melzer, D., 'Genetics and medicalisation', *British Medical Journal*, 2002, vol. 321: 863–64

16 Finch, C.E., Tanzi, R.E., 'Genetics of aging', *Science*, 1997, vol. 278: 407–11

17 Svendsen, J. et al., 'Relative importance of genetic effects in rheumatoid arthritis: Historical cohort study of Danish nationwide twin population', *British Medical Journal*, 2002, vol. 324: 264–66

18 Begg, C.B., 'On the use of familial aggregation in population-based case probands for calculating penetrance', *Journal of the National Cancer Institute*, 2002, vol. 94: 1221–26; Haffty, B.G. et al., 'Outcome of conservatively managed early-onset breast cancer by BRCA1/2 status', *The Lancet*, 2002, vol. 359: 1471–77

19 Boutin, P. et al., 'GAD2 on chromosome 10p12 is a candidate gene for human obesity', *Public Library of Science Biology*, 2003, vol. 1 (3): e68.doi:10.1371/journal.pbio.0000068

20 Waldenmaier, B. et al., 'Lack of support for the association between GAD2 polymorphisms and severe human obesity, *Public Library of Science Biology*, 2005, vol. 3 (9): e315 doi:10.1371/journal.pbio.0030315

21 Walston, J. et al., 'Time of onset of non-insulin-dependent diabetes mellitus and genetic variation in the b3-adrenergic receptor gene', *New England Journal of Medicine*, 1995, vol. 333: 343–47; Widen, E. et al., 'Association of a polymorphism in the b3-adrenergic receptor gene with features of the insulin resistance syndrome in Finns', *New England Journal of Medicine*, 1995, vol. 333: 348–51; Clement, K. et al., 'Genetic variation in the b3-adrenergic receptor and an increased capacity to gain weight in patients with morbid obesity', *New England Journal of Medicine*, 1995, vol. 333: 352–54; see also Arner, P., 'The b-3-adrenergic receptor – a cause and cure of obesity?', *New England Journal of Medicine*, 1995, vol. 333: 382–83

22 Frayling, T.M. et al., 'A common variant in the FTO gene is associated with body mass index and predisposes to childhood and adult obesity', *Science*, 12 April 2007, DOI: 10.1126/science.1141634

23 Stunkard, A.J. et al., 'An adoption study of human obesity', *New England Journal of Medicine*, 1986, vol. 314:193–98

24 Mishmar, D. et al., 'Natural selection shaped regional mtDNA variation in humans', *Proceedings of the National Academy of Sciences*, 2003, vol. 100: 171–76

25 Keith, S.W. et al., 'Putative contributors to the secular increase in obesity: Exploring the roads less travelled', *International Journal of Obesity*, advance online publication, 27 June 2006, doi:10.1038/sj.ijo.0803326

Chapter 3: Sleep yourself thin

1 Ayas, N.T. et al., 'A prospective study of sleep duration and coronary heart disease in women', *Archives of Internal Medicine*, 2003, vol. 163: 205–09

2 Boethel, C.D., 'Sleep and the endocrine system: New associations to old diseases', *Current Opinion in Pulmonary Medicine*, 2002, vol. 8: 502–05

3 Currie, A., Cappuccio, F.P., 'Sleep in children and adolescents: A worrying scenario', *Nutrition, Metabolism & Cardiovascular Diseases*, 2007, vol. 17: 230–32

4 Heymsfield, S., Gangwisch, J., 'Deprivation as a risk factor for obesity: Results based on the NHANES I', Paper presented at the annual meeting of the North American Association for the Study of Obesity, Las Vegas, November 2004

5 Vorona, R.D. et al., 'Overweight and obese patients in a primary care population report less sleep than patients with a normal body mass index', *Archives of Internal Medicine*, 2005, vol. 165: 25–30; Bass, J., Turek, F.W., 'Sleepless in America: A pathway to obesity and the metabolic syndrome?', *Archives of Internal Medicine*, 2005, vol. 165: 15–16

6 Kripke, D.F. et al., 'Mortality associated with sleep duration and insomnia', *Archives of General Psychiatry*, 2002, vol. 59: 131–36

7 Hasler, G. et al., 'The association between short sleep duration and obesity in young adults: A 13-Year Prospective Study', *Sleep*, 2004, vol. 27 (4): 661–65

8 Sekine, M. et al., 'A dose–response relationship between short sleeping hours and childhood obesity: Results of the Toyama Birth Cohort Study', *Child: Care, Health and Development*, 2002, vol. 28 (2): 163–70

9 Vioque, J. et al., 'Time spent watching television, sleep duration and obesity in adults living in Valencia, Spain', *International Journal of Obesity-Related Metabolic Disorders*, 2000, vol. 24: 1683–88

10 Locard, E. et al., 'Risk factors of obesity in a five-year-old population: Parental versus environmental factors', *International Journal of Obesity-Related Metabolic Disorders*, 1992, vol. 16: 721–29

11 Gupta, N.K., Mueller, W.H., Chan, W., Meininger, J.C., 'Is

obesity associated with poor sleep quality in adolescents?', *American Journal of Human Biology*, 2002, vol. 14: 762–68

12 Owens, J., Maxim, R., McGuinn, M., Nobile, C., Msall, M., Alario, A., 'Television-viewing habits and sleep disturbance in school children', *Pediatrics*, 1999, vol. 104: e27

13 Ibid., vol. 104 (3); Johnson, J.G., Cohen, P., Kasen, S., First, M.B., Brook, J.S., 'Association between television viewing and sleep problems during adolescence and early adulthood', *Archives of Pediatrics & Adolescent Medicine*, 2004, vol. 158: 562–68

14 Higuchi, S., Motohashi, Y., Liu, Y., Ahara, M., Kaneko, Y., 'Effects of VDT tasks with a bright display at night on melatonin, core temperature, heart rate, and sleepiness', *Journal of Applied Physiology*, 2003, vol. 94: 1773–76; Kubota, T., Uchiyama, M., Suzuki, H. et al., 'Effects of nocturnal bright light on saliva melatonin, core body temperature and sleep propensity rhythms in human subjects', *Neuroscience Research*, 2002, vol. 42: 115–22

15 Sheen, A.J. et al., 'Relationships between sleep quality and glucose regulation in normal humans', *American Journal of Physiology*, 1996, vol. 271 (2 Pt 1): E261–70

16 Van Cauter, E. et al., 'Modulation of glucose regulation and insulin secretion by circadian rhythmicity and sleep', *Journal of Clinical Investigation*, 1991, vol. 88: 934–42

17 Spiegel, K. et al., 'Impact of sleep debt on metabolic and endocrine function', *The Lancet*, 1999, vol. 354: 1435–39

18 Taheri, S. et al., 'Short sleep duration is associated with reduced leptin, elevated ghrelin, and increased body mass index', *Public Library of Science Medicine*, 2004, vol. 1 (3): 210–17

19 Ayas, N.T. et al., 'A prospective study of self-reported sleep duration and incident diabetes in women', *Diabetes Care*, 2003, vol. 26: 380–84

20 Coy, T.V. et al., 'The role of sleep-disordered breathing in essential hypertension', *Chest*, 1996, vol. 109 (4): 890–95; Iyer, S.R., Iyer, R.R., 'Sleep and obesity in the causation of metabolic syndrome', *International Journal of Diabetes in Developing Countries*, 2006, vol. 26: 63–69

21 Hunsaker, D.H., Riffenburgh, R.H., 'Snoring significance in patients undergoing home sleep studies', *Archives of Otolaryngology – Head & Neck Surgery*, May 2006, vol. 134 (5): 756–60

22 Strohl, K.P., Boehm, K.D., Denko, C.W. et al., 'Biochemical morbidity in sleep apnoea', *ENT Journal*, 1993, vol. 72 (1): 38–41; Fletcher, E., 'The relationship between systemic hypertension and obstructive sleep apnoea: Facts and theory', *American Journal of Medicine*, 1995, vol. 98: 118–28; Stradling, J.R. et al., 'Effect of short-term, graded withdrawal of nasal continuous positive airway pressure on systemic blood pressure in patients with obstructive sleep apnoea', *Blood Pressure*, 1996, vol. 5 (4): 234–40; Ziegler, M.G. et al., 'Sleep apnoea, norepinephrine-release rate and daytime hypertension', *Sleep*, 1997, vol. 20 (3): 224–31

23 'Sleep could be key to weight management', Findings at Baylor College, University of Texas, October 2003, vol. 1, issue 10

24 'Short sleep duration is associated with reduced leptin levels and increased body weight: Results', Paper presented to the 2005 Annual Scientific Meeting of NAASO, The Obesity Society, Vancouver, 18 October 2005

25 Morse, D.R. et al., 'A physiological and subjective evaluation of meditation, hypnosis, and relaxation', *Psychosomatic Medicine*, 1977, vol. 39: 304–24; Morse, D.R. et al., 'Physiological responses during meditation and rest', *Biofeedback & Self Regulation*, 1984, vol. 9: 181–200

26 Schneider, R.H. et al., 'A randomised controlled trial of stress reduction for hypertension in older African Americans', *Hypertension*, 1995, vol. 26: 820–27; Schneider, R.H. et al., 'Lower lipid peroxide levels in practitioners of the Transcendental Meditation program', *Psychosomatic Medicine*, 1998, vol. 60: 38–41; Ornish, D. et al., 'Can lifestyle changes reverse atherosclerosis?', *The Lancet*, 1990, vol. 336: 129–33; Gould, K.L. et al., 'Changes in myocardial perfusion abnormalities by positron emission tomography after long-term, intense risk factor modification', *Journal of the American Medical Association*, 1995, vol. 27: 894–901; Gould, K.L. et al., 'Improved stenosis geometry by quantitative coronary arteriography after vigorous risk factor modification', *American Journal of Cardiology*, 1992, vol. 69: 845–53

27 Glaser, J.L. et al., 'Elevated serum dehydroepiandrosterone sulfate levels in practitioners of the Transcendental Meditation (TM) and TM-Sidhi programs', *Journal of Behavioral Medicine*, 1992, vol. 15: 327–41

28 Kaplan, K.H. et al., 'The impact of a meditation-based stress reduction program on fibromyalgia', *General Hospital Psychiatry*, 1993, vol. 15: 284–89; Taylor, D.N., 'Effects of a behavioral stress-management program on anxiety, mood, self-esteem and T-cell count in HIV positive men', *Psychological Reports*, 1995, vol. 76: 451–57

29 Hahn, R.A., 'Profound bilateral blindness and the incidence of breast cancer', *Epidemiology*, 1991, vol. 2: 208–10; Coleman, M.P., Reiter, R.J., 'Breast cancer, blindness and melatonin', *European Journal of Cancer*, 1992, vol. 28: 501–03; Kliukiene, J., Tynes, T., Andersen, A., 'Risk of breast cancer among Norwegian women with visual impairment', *British Journal of Cancer*, 2001, vol. 84: 397–99

30 Feychting, M. et al., 'Reduced cancer incidence among the

blind', *Epidemiology*, 1998, vol. 9: 490–94; Verkasalo, P.K. et al., 'Inverse association between breast cancer incidence and degree of visual impairment in Finland', *British Journal of Cancer*, 1999, vol. 80: 1459–60

Chapter 4: The problem of 'chemical calories'

1 Walford, R., 'Physiologic changes in humans subjected to severe, selective calorie restriction for two years in biosphere 2: Health, aging and toxicological perspectives', *Toxicological Sciences*, 1999, vol. 52: 61–65

2 Mead, N.M., 'Origins of obesity: Chemical exposures', *Environmental Health Perspectives*, May 2004, vol. 112 (6): A344

3 Baillie-Hamilton, P., 'Chemical toxins: A hypothesis to explain the global obesity epidemic', *Journal of Alternative & Complementary Medicine*, 2002, vol. 8: 185–92

4 Thomas, P., 'The big fat fix', *The Ecologist*, September 2006, 33–43

5 Backman, L., Kolmodin-Hedman, B., 'Concentration of DDT and DDE in plasma and subcutaneous adipose tissue before and after intestinal bypass operation for treatment of obesity', *Toxicology and Applied Pharmacology*, 1978, vol. 46: 663–69

6 Pelletier, C. et al., 'Association between weight loss-induced changes in plasma organochlorine concentrations, serum T(3) concentration and resting metabolic rate', *Toxicological Sciences*, 2002, 67 (1): 46–51; also Imbeault, P. et al., 'Weight loss induced rise in plasma pollutant is associated with reduced skeletal muscle oxidative capacity', *American Journal of Physiology – Endocrinology and Metabolism*, 2002, vol. 282: E574–79

7 Tremblay, A. et al., 'Thermogenesis and weight loss in obese individuals: A primary association with organochlorine

pollution', *International Journal of Obesity*, 2004, vol. 28 (July): 936–39

8 Masumo, H. et al., 'Bisphenol A in combination with insulin can accelerate the conversion of 3T3L1 fibroblasts into adipocytes', *Journal of Lipid Research*, 2002, vol. 43: 676–84; also Grun, F., Blumberg, B., 'Environmental obesogens: Organotins and endocrine disruption via nuclear receptor signalling', *Endocrinology*, June 2006, vol. 147 (6 supplement): S50–55

9 Michalek, J.E., Tripathi, R.C., 'Pharmacokinetics of TCDD in veterans of operation ranch hand: 15-year follow-up', *Journal of Toxicology and Environmental Health*, 1999, vol. 57: 369–78

10 Pelletier, C. et al., 'Energy Balance and pollution by organochlorines and polychlorinated biphenyls', *Obesity Reviews*, 2003, vol. 4 (1): 17–24

11 Breslin, W.J., Liberacki, A.B., Dittenber, D.A., Quast, J.F., 'Evaluation of the developmental and reproductive toxicity of chlorpyrifos in the rat', *Fundamental and Applied Toxicology*, 1996, vol. 29 (1): 119-30; also Nicolau, G.Y., 'Circadian rhythms of RNA, DNA and protein in the rat thyroid, adrenal and testis in chronic pesticide exposure: III. Effects of the insecticides (dichlorvos and trichlorphon)', *Physiologie*, 1983, vol. 20 (2): 93–101

12 Walker, E.M. et al., 'Prevention of cis-platin-induced toxicology by selected dithiocarbamates', *Annals of Clinical and Laboratory Science*, 1994, vol. 24 (2): 121–33; also Yen, J.T. et al., 'Effect of carbadox on growth, fasting metabolism, thyroid function and gastrointestinal tract in young pigs', *Journal of Nutrition*, 1984, vol. 115: 970–79

13 Grun, F., Blumberg, B., 'Environmental obesogens: Organotins and endocrine disruption via nuclear receptor signalling', *Endocrinology*, June 2006, vol. 147 (6 supplement): S5055

14 Masumo, H. et al., 'Bisphenol A in combination with insulin can accelerate the conversion of 3T3L1 fibroblasts into adipocytes', *Journal of Lipid Research*, 2002, vol. 43: 676–84; also Howdeshell, K.L. et al., 'Exposure to bisphenol A advances puberty', *Nature*, 1999, vol. 401 (6755): 763–64

15 Lamb, J.C. et al., 'Reproductive effects of four phthalic acid esters in the mouse', *Toxicology and Applied Pharmacology*, 1987, vol. 88 (2): 255–69; also Field, E.A. et al., 'Developmental toxicology evaluation of diethyl and dimethyl phthalate in rats', *Teratology*, 1993, vol. 48 (1): 33–44

16 Gupta, B.N. et al., 'Effects of a polybrominated biphenyl mixture in the rat and mouse: I. Six-month exposure', *Toxicology and Applied Pharmacology*, 1983, vol. 68 (1): 1–18

17 Irigaray, P. et al., 'Benzo[a]pyrene impairs b-adrenergeti stimulation of adipose tissue lipolysis and causes weight gain in mice', *FEBS Journal*, 2006, vol. 273: 1362–72

18 Moser, V.C. et al., 'A multidisciplinary approach to toxicological screening: III. Neurobehavioural toxicology', *Journal of Toxicology and Environmental Health*, 1995, vol. 45 (2): 173–210; also Hardin, B. et al., 'Evaluation of 60 chemicals in a preliminary developmental toxicity test', *Teratogenesis, Carcinogenesis and Mutagenesis*, 1987, vol. 7 (1): 29–48; also Wahlberg, J.E., Boman, A., 'Comparative percutaneous toxicity of ten industrial solvents in the guinea pig', *Scandinavian Journal of Work, Environment & Health*, 1979, vol. 5 (4): 345–51

19 Antonio, M.T. et al., 'Neurochemical changes in newborn rat's brain after gestational cadmium and lead exposure', *Toxicology Letters*, 1999, vol. 104 (1–2): 1–9

20 Hovinga, M.E. et al., 'Environmental exposure and lifestyle predictors of lead, cadmium, PCB, and DDT levels in great lakes fish eaters', *Archives of Environmental Health*, 1993, vol. 48: 98–104

21 Hawkes, N., 'Fat map pinpoints the streets with a weight problem', *The Times*, 1 September 2006

22 *F as in Fat 2006: How Obesity Policies are Failing in America*, Trust for America's Health, 2006

23 US Environmental Protection Agency (EPA), Toxic Release Inventory, 1990–1994

24 EPA, Toxic Release Inventory, 2004

25 Calle, E.E. et al., 'Cigarette smoking and risk of fatal breast cancer', *American Journal of Epidemiology*, 1994, vol. 139: 1001–07

26 Roberts, R.J., 'Overview of similarities and differences between children and adults: Implications for risk assessment', in Guzelian, P.S. et al. (eds), *Similarities and Differences Between Children and Adults*, ILSI Press, 1992: 1–15

27 Bearer, C.F., 'How are children different from adults?', *Environmental Health Perspectives*, 1995, vol. 103 (supplement 6): 7–12

28 Rogers, S.A., 'Diagnosing the sick building syndrome', *Environmental Health Perspectives*, 1987, vol. 76: 195–98; Godish, T., *Sick Buildings: Definition, Diagnosis and Mitigation*, Lewis Publications, 1995

29 Cullen, M.R., 'Workers with multiple chemical sensitivity', *Occupational Medicine*, 1987, vol. 2: 655–61; Hileman, B., 'Multiple chemical sensitivity', *Chemical & Engineering News*, 1991, vol. 69: 26–42; Rea, W.J., *Chemical Sensitivity*, vols 1, 2, 3, Lewis Publications, 1992, 1994, 1996

30 Crinnion, W.J., 'Environmental medicine, Part 1: The human burden of environmental toxins and their common health effects', *Alternative Medicine Review*, 2000, vol. 5: 52–63

31 Ashford, N.A., Miller, C.S., *Chemical Exposures: Low Levels and High Stakes*, Van Nostrand Reinhold, 1991

32 Randolph, T., *Human Ecology and Susceptibility to the*

Chemical Environment, Charles C. Thomas, 1962; Randolph, T., *Environmental Medicine – Beginnings and Bibliography of Clinical Ecology*, Clinical Ecology Publications, 1987

33 Schettler, T. et al., *In Harm's Way: Toxic Threats to Child Development*, Greater Boston Physicians for Social Responsibility, June 2000

34 Biles, J.E. et al., 'Determination of bisphenol A in re-usable polycarbonate food contact plastics and migration to food-simulating liquids', *Journal of Agriculture and Food Chemistry*, 1997, vol. 45: 3541–4; Lambert, C., Larroque, M., 'Chromatographic analysis of water and wine samples for phenolic compounds released from food contact expoxy resins', *Journal of Chromatographic Science*, 1997, vol. 35: 57–62

35 Brotons, J.A. et al., 'Xenoestrogens released from lacquer coatings in food cans', *Environmental Health Perspectives*, 1995, vol. 103: 608–12

36 Yoshida, T. et al., 'Determination of bisphenol A in canned vegetables and fruit by high performance liquid chromatography', *Food Additives and Contaminants*, 2001, vol. 18: 69–75

37 Barrett, J.R., 'Soy and children's health: A formula for trouble', *Environmental Health Perspectives*, 2002, vol. 110: A294–96

38 Strom, B.L., 'Exposure to soy-based formula in infancy and endocrinological and reproductive outcomes in young adulthood', *Journal of the American Medical Association*, 2001, vol. 286: 807–14

39 Eklund, G., Oskarsson, A., 'Exposure of cadmium from infant formulas and weaning foods', *Food Additives and Contaminants*, 1999, vol. 16: 509–19

40 Worldwide Fund for Nature, *Bisphenol A – A Known Endocrine Disruptor, A WWF European Toxics Programme*

Report, April 2000

41 Santodonato, J., 'Review of the estrogenic and antiestrogenic activity of polycyclic aromatic hydrocarbons: Relationship to carcinogenicity', *Chemosphere*, 1997, vol. 34: 835–48; Arcaro, K.F. et al., 'Antiestrogenicity of environmental polycyclic aromatic hydrocarbons in human breast cancer cells', *Toxicology*, 1999, vol. 133: 115–27

42 Routledge, E.J. et al., 'Some alkyl hydroxy benzoate preservatives (parabens) are estrogenic', *Toxicology and Applied Pharmacology*, 1998, vol. 153: 12–19

43 Schlumpf, M. et al., 'In vitro and in vivo estrogenicity of UV screens', *Environmental Health Perspectives*, 2001, vol. 109: 239–44; Nakagawa, Y. et al., 'Metabolism and toxicity of benzophenone in isolated rat hepatocytes and estrogenic activity of its metabolites in MCF-7 cells', *Toxicology*, 2000, vol. 156: 27–36

44 Ford, R.A. et al., '90-day dermal toxicity study and neurotoxicity evaluation of nitromusks in the albino rat', *Food and Chemical Toxicology*, 1990, vol. 28: 55–56

45 Geldof, A.A. et al., 'Estrogenic action of commonly used fragrant agent citral induces prostatic hyperplasia', *Urology Research*, 1992, vol. 20: 139–44

46 Sharma-Wagner, S. et al., 'Occupation and prostate cancer risk in Sweden', *Journal of Occupational and Environmental Medicine*, 2000, vol. 42: 517–25

47 Seinen, W. et al., 'AHTN and HHCB show weak estrogenic – but no uterotrophic activity', *Toxicology Letters*, 1999, vol. 111: 161–68; Blount, B.C. et al., 'Levels of seven urinary phthalate metabolites in a human reference population', *Environmental Health Perspectives*, 2000, vol. 108: 979–82

48 Environmental Health Network of California, *FDA Petition no. 99P-1340*, filed May 1999

49 Ilonka, A. et al., 'Potent competitive interactions of some brominated flame retardants and related compounds with human transthyretin in vitro', *Toxicological Sciences*, 2000, vol. 56: 95–104

50 Rea, W.J. et al., 'Clearing of toxic volatile hydrocarbons from humans', *Boletín de la Asociación Médica de Puerto Rico*, 1991, vol. 83: 321–24; Kilburn, K.H. et al., 'Neurobehavioral dysfunction in firemen exposed to polychlorinated biphenyls (PCBs): Possible improvement after detoxification', *Archives of Environmental Health*, 1989, vol. 44: 345–50; Tretjak, Z. et al., 'PCB reduction and clinical improvement by detoxification: An unexploited approach?', *Human and Experimental Toxicology*, 1990, vol. 9: 235–44

51 Czarnowski, D., Gorski, J., 'Excretion of nitrogen compounds in sweat during a sauna', *Polski tygodnik lekarski*, 1991, vol. 46: 186–87

52 Kroker, G.A. et al., 'Fasting and rheumatoid arthritis: A multicenter study', *Clinical Ecology*, 1984, vol. 3: 137–44; Kjeldsen-Kragh, J. et al., 'Controlled trial of fasting and one-year vegetarian diet in rheumatoid arthritis', *The Lancet*, 1991, vol. 338: 899–902; Skoldstam, L. et al., 'Effects of fasting and lactovegetarian diet on rheumatoid arthritis', *Scandinavian Journal of Rheumatology*, 1979, vol. 8; 249–55; Lithell, H. et al., 'A fasting and vegetarian diet treatment trial on chronic inflammatory disorders', *Acta Dermato-Venereologica*, 1983, vol. 63: 397–403

53 Duncan, T.G. et al., 'Contraindications and therapeutic results of fasting in obese patients', *Annals of the New York Academy of Sciences*, 1965, vol. 131: 632–36; Gresham, G.A., 'Is atheroma a reversible lesion?', *Atherosclerosis*, 1976, vol. 23: 379–91; Maislos, M. et al., 'Gorging and plasma HDL-cholesterol – the Ramadan model', *European Journal of Clinical*

Nutrition, 1998, vol. 52: 127–30

54 Navarro, S. et al., 'Comparison of fasting, nasogastric suction and cimetidine in treatment of acute pancreatitis', *Digestion*, 1984, vol. 30: 224–30

55 Boheme, D.L. 'Preplanned fasting in the treatment of mental disease: Survey of the current Soviet literature', *Schizophrenia Bulletin*, 1977, vol. 3: 288–96

56 Imamura, M., Tung, T., 'A trial of fasting cure for PCB poisoned patients in Taiwan', *American Journal of Industrial Medicine*, 1984, vol. 5: 147–53

57 Haas, E., *The Detox Diet*, Celestial Arts, 1996: 115

58 Perical, M., Percival, S., *Infant Nutrition*, Health Coach Systems International, 1995

Chapter 5: Pills that make you plump

1 Dobson, R., 'Huge weight gains reported by patients on prescription drugs', *The Independent on Sunday*, 24 June 2007

2 Leslie, W.S. et al., 'Weight gain as an adverse effect of some commonly prescribed drugs: A systematic review', *Quarterly Journal of Medicine*, advance online publication, 12 June 2007; doi:10.1093/qjmed/hcm044

3 Kulkarni, S.K., Kaur, G., 'Pharmacodynamics of drug-induced weight gain', *Drugs Today*, 2001, vol. 37 (8): 559–72

4 Hays, V.W., 'Effect of Antibiotics', in Pearson, A.M., Dutson, T.R. (eds), *Growth Regulation in Farm Animals*, Elsevier Applied Science, 1999: 299–320

5 National Institute for Clinical Excellence, *The Treatment of Depression in Primary and Secondary Care*, 2004, NICE

6 Rose, D., 'Britain becomes a Prozac nation', *The Times*, 14 May 2007

7 Stagnitti, M., *Antidepressant Use in the US Civilian Non-*

Institutionalised Population, 2002. Statistical Brief #77, Medical Expenditure Panel, Agency for Healthcare Research and Quality, 2005

8 Burt, C.W. et al., 'Ambulatory Medical Care Utilization Estimates for 2005', 29 June 2007; online at: *www.cdc. gov/nchs/data/ad/ad388.pdf*

9 Vedantam, S., 'Antidepressant use in children soars despite efficacy doubts', *Washington Post*, 18 April 2004: A01

10 Masand, P.S., 'Weight gain associated with psychotropic drugs', *Expert Opinion on Pharmacotherapy* 2000, vol. 1 (3): 377–89; Ruetsch, O. et al., 'Psychotropic drugs induced weight gain: A review of the literature concerning epidemiological data, mechanisms and management', *Encephale*, 2005, vol. 31 (4 Pt 1): 507–16; Fava, M., 'Weight gain and antidepressants', *Journal of Clinical Psychiatry*, 2006, vol. 61 (supplement 11): 37–41

11 Olfson, M. et al., 'National trends in the outpatient treatment of children and adolescents with antipsychotic drugs', *Archives of General Psychiatry*, 2006, vol. 63: 679–85

12 Allison, D.B. et al., 'Antipsychotic-induced weight gain: A comprehensive research synthesis', *American Journal of Psychiatry*, 1999, vol. 156: 1686–96

13 National Institute for Clinical Excellence, *Clinical Guideline 18 – Management of hypertension in adults in primary care*, 2004, NICE; see also Mason, J.M. et al., 'The diabetogenic potential of thiazide-type diuretic and beta-blocker combinations in patients with hypertension', *Journal of Hypertension*, 2005, vol. 3: 1777–81

14 Sharma, A.M. et al., 'Hypothesis: Beta-adrenergic receptor blockers and weight gain: A systematic analysis', *Hypertension*, 2001, vol. 37 (2): 250–54

15 Wilding, J., 'Thiazolidinediones, insulin resistance and obesity: Finding a balance', *International Journal of Clinical*

Practice, 2006, vol. 60 (10): 1272–80

16 Martens, F.M. et al., 'Metabolic and additional vascular effects of thiazolidinediones', *Drugs*, 2002, vol. 62: 1463–80; Lebovitz, H.E., 'Differentiating members of the thiazolidinedione class: A focus on safety', *Diabetes/Metabolism Research and Reviews*, 2002, vol. 18 (supplement 2): S23–29; Barnett, A.H., 'Insulin-sensitizing agents – thiazolidinediones (glitazones)', *Current Medical Research and Opinion*, 2002, vol. 18 (supplement 1): S31–39; Scheen, A.J., 'Glitazones and weight gain', *Annals of Endocrinology* (Paris), 2002, vol. 63: IS412–14

17 Purnell, J.Q., Weyer, C., 'Weight effect of current and experimental drugs for diabetes mellitus: From promotion to alleviation of obesity', *Treatments in Endocrinology*, 2003, vol. 2 (1): 33–47

18 Diabetes Control and Complications Trial Research Group, 'The effect of intensive treatment of diabetes on the development and progression of long-term complications in insulin-dependent diabetes mellitus', *New England Journal of Medicine*, 1993, vol. 329: 977–86

19 UK Prospective Diabetes Study (UKPDS) Group, 'Intensive blood-glucose control with sulphonylureas or insulin compared with conventional treatment and risk of complications in patients with type 2 diabetes (UKPDS 33)', *The Lancet*, 1998, vol. 352: 837–53

20 Raskin, P. et al., 'A randomized trial of rosiglitazone therapy in patients with inadequately controlled insulin-treated type 2 diabetes', *Diabetes Care*, 2001, vol. 24: 1226–32

21 Adams, M. et al., 'Activators of peroxisome proliferator-activated receptor y have depot-specific effects on human preadipocyte differentiation', *Journal of Clinical Investigation*, 1997, vol. 100: 3149–53

22 Arares, M. et al., 'Estrogen-induced weight gain cannot be predicted in individuals', *Klinische Wochenschrift*, 1986, vol. 64

(13): 623–24

23 Petersen, K.R. et al., 'Metabolic and fibrinolytic response to changed insulin sensitivity in users of oral contraceptives', *Contraception*, 1999, vol. 60 (6): 337–44; Sheu, W.H. et al., 'Prospective evaluation of insulin resistance and lipid metabolism in women receiving oral contraceptives', *Clinical Endocrinology (Oxford)*, 1994, vol. 40 (2): 249–55

24 Vigano, A., 'Anorexia and cachexia in advanced cancer patients', *Cancer Surveys*, 1994, vol. 21: 99–115

25 *House of Lords Committee Report, Science and Technology*, seventh edition, 1998, chapter 12.5, paragraph 11.18

26 Young, R., Craig, A., *Use and Misuse of Antibiotics in UK Agriculture, Part 3: Too hard to swallow: the truth about drugs and poultry*, Soil Association, 4 June 2001

27 Hughes, P., Heritage, J., 'Antibiotics growth promoters in food animals', FAO Animal and Health Promotion Paper, 2004, vol. 160: 129–52; online at: *www.fao.org/DOCREP/ARTICLE/AGRIPPA/555_EN.HTM*

28 Nesheim, M.C., 'Some observations on the effectiveness of anabolic agents in increasing the growth rate of poultry', *Environmental Quality and Safety*, 1976 (supplement), vol. 5: 110–14

29 Zwick, D., *Water Wasteland: Ralph Nader's Study Group Report on Water Pollution*, Viking Press, 1971

30 Barbash, J.E., Resek, E.A., *Pesticides in Ground Water*, Ann Arbor Press, 1996; Cohen, B.A., Wiles, R., *Tough to Swallow*, Environmental Working Group, 1997; Environmental Working Group, *Pouring it On: Nitrate Contamination of Drinking Water*, Environmental Working Group, 1996; Solomon, G.M., Mott, L., *Trouble on the Farm: Growing Up With Pesticides in Agricultural Communities*, Natural Resources Defense Council, October 1998

31 'What are the health effects of contaminants in drinking water?', EPA Office of Water; online at: *www.epa.gov/ safewater/dwh/health.html*

32 Hignite, C., Azarnoff, D.L., 'Drugs and drug metabolites as environmental contaminants: Chlorophenoxyisobutyrate and salicyclic acid in sewage water effluent', *Life Sciences*, 1977, vol. 20: 337–41

33 Daughton, C.G., Ternes, T.A., 'Pharmaceuticals and personal care products in the environment: Agents of subtle change', *Environmental Health Perspectives*, 1999, vol. 107 (supplement 6): 907–38; Raloff, J., 'Drugged waters', *Science News*, 1998, vol. 153: 187–89

34 Buser, H.R., Muller, M.D., 'Occurrence of the pharmaceutical drug clofibric acid and the herbicide mecoprop in various Swiss lakes and in the North Sea', *Environmental Science & Technology*, 1998, vol. 32: 188–92

35 US Geological Society (US) [USGS], 'Pharmaceuticals, hormones, and other organic wastewater contaminants in US streams', June 2002; online at: *http://toxics.usgs.gov/pubs/FS-027-02/*

36 Stackelberg, P.E. et al., 'Persistence of pharmaceutical compounds and other organic wastewater contaminants in a conventional drinking-water-treatment plant', *Science of the Total Environment*, 2004, vol. 329 (1–3): 99–113

37 *Review of Human Pharmaceuticals in the Environment, Research and Development Technical Report P390*, Environment Agency, 2003

38 Hancock, J.F., 'Effects of estrogens and androgens on animal growth', in Pearson, A.M., Dutson, T.R. (ed.), *Growth Regulation in Farm Animals*, Elsevier Scientific Publications Ltd: 225

39 Andelman, J.B., 'Human exposures to volatile halogenated organic chemicals in indoor and outdoor air', *Environmental Health Perspectives*, 1985, vol. 62: 313–18

40 Brown, H.S. et al., 'The role of skin absorption as a route of exposure for volatile organic compounds (VOCs) in drinking water', *American Journal of Public Health*, 1984, vol. 74: 479–84; Maxwell, N.I. et al., 'Trihalomethanes and maximum contaminant levels: The significance of inhalation and dermal exposures to chloroform in household water', *Regulatory Toxicology and Pharmacology*, 1991, vol. 14: 297–312; Jo, W.K. et al., 'Routes of chloroform exposure and body burden from showering with chlorinated tap water', *Risk Analysis*, 1990, vol. 10: 575–80

41 Potera, C., 'Our drugged drinking water', *Environmental Health Perspectives*, 2000, vol. 108 (10): A446

42 Kidd, K.A. et al., 'Collapse of a fish population after exposure to a synthetic estrogen', *Proceedings of the National Academy of Sciences*, 2007, vol. 104 (21): 8897–901

43 Raloff, J., 'Waterways carry antibiotic resistance', *Science News Online*, 5 June 1999; online at: *www.sciencenews.org/ sn_arc99/6_5_99/fob1.htm*

Chapter 6: The influence of allergies

1 Scientic Committee On Consumer Products, *Fragrance Allergy in Consumers: A Review of the Problem. Analysis of the need for appropriate consumer information and identification of consumer allergens*, 1999

2 Wilson, B.G., Bahna, S.L., 'Adverse reactions of food additives', *Annals of Allergy, Asthma & Immunology*, 2005, vol. 95: 499–507; Bush, R.K. et al., 'Adverse reactions to food and drug additives', in Adkinson, N.F., Yunginger, J.W., Busse, W.W. et al. (eds), *Middleton's Allergy Principles and Practice*, 6th edition, Mosby Publishing, 2003: 1645–63

3 Bates, C.E., *Beyond Dieting: Relief from Persistent Hunger*, Tsolum River Press, 1994

4 Breneman, J.C., *Basics of Food Allergy*, Charles C. Thomas, 1978

5 D'Adamo, P., Whitney, C., *Eat Right 4 Your Type*, G.P. Putnam's Sons, 1996; D'Adamo, P., Whitney, C., *Allergies: Fight Them with the Blood Type Diet*, G.P. Putnam's Sons, 2005

6 Nachbar, M.S., Oppenheim, J.D., 'Lectins in the United States diet: A survey of lectins in commonly consumed foods and a review of the literature', *American Journal of Clinical Nutrition*, 1980, vol. 33: 2338–45; see also D'Adamo, J., *One Man's Food is Someone Else's Poison*, Marek, 1980

7 Mozaf Tarian, D. et al., 'Dietary intake of trans fatty acids and systemic inflammation in women', *American Journal of Clinical Nutrition*, 2004, vol. 79 (4): 606–12; Lopez-Garcia, E. et al., 'Consumption of trans fatty acids is related to plasma biomarkers of inflammation and endothelial dysfunction', *Journal of Nutrition*, 2005, vol. 135 (3): 562–66; Liu, S. et al., 'Relation between a diet with a high glycemic load and plasma concentrations of high-sensitivity C-reactive protein in middle-aged women', *American Journal of Clinical Nutrition*, 2002, vol. 75 (3): 492–98

8 Balagopal, P. et al., 'Lifestyle-only intervention attenuates the inflammatory state associated with obesity: A randomized controlled study in adolescents', *Journal of Pediatrics*, 2005, vol. 146: 342–48

9 Seematter, G. et al., 'Relationship between stress, inflammation and metabolism', *Current Opinion in Clinical Nutrition and Metabolic Care*, March 2004, vol. 7 (2): 169–73; Black, P.H., 'The inflammatory response is an integral part of the stress response: Implications for atherosclerosis, insulin resistance, type

II diabetes and metabolic syndrome X', *Brain, Behavior, and Immunity*, 2003, vol. 17 (5): 3SO-64

10 Girard, D., 'Activation of human polymorphonuclear neutrophils by environmental contaminants', *Review of Environmental Health*, 2003, vol. 18 (2): 75–89; Pelletier, M. et al., 'Activation of human neutrophils in vitro and dieldrin-induced neutrophilic inflammation in vivo', *Journal of Leucocyte Biology*, 2001, vol. 70 (3): S67–73

11 Alexander, W.S., Hilton, D.J., 'The role of suppressors of cytokine signaling (SOCS) proteins in regulation of the immune response', *Annual Review of Immunology*, 2004, vol. 22: 503–29; Elliott, J., Johnston, J.A., 'SOCS: Role in inflammation, allergy and homeostasis', *Trends in Immunology*, 2004, vol. 25 (8): 434–40; Serhan, C.N., 'A search for endogenous mechanisms of anti-inflammation uncovers novel chemical mediators: Missing links to resolution', *Histochemistry and Cell Biology*, 2004, vol. 122 (4): 305–21

12 Galland, L., *The Fat Resistance Diet*, Broadway Books, 2006

13 Das, U.N., 'Is obesity an inflammatory condition?', *Nutrition*, 2001, vol. 17 (11–12): 953-G6

14 Ferroni, P. et al., 'Inflammation, insulin resistance, and obesity', *Current Atherosclerosis Reports*, 2004, vol. 6 (6): 424–31; Sonnenberg, G.E. et al., 'A novel pathway to the manifestations of metabolic syndrome', *Obesity Research*, February 2004, vol. 12 (2): 180–86; Grimble, R.F., 'Inflammatory status and insulin resistance', *Current Opinion in Clinical Nutrition and Metabolic Care*, 2002, vol. 5 (5): 551–59; Moller, D.E., 'Potential role of TNF-alpha in the patho-genesis of insulin resistance and type 2 diabetes', *Trends in Endocrinology and Metabolism*, 2000, vol. 11 (6): 212–17

15 Skurk, T. et al., 'Production and release of macrophage migration inhibitory factor from human adipocytes',

Endocrinology, 2005, vol. 146 (s): 1006–11; Weisberg, S.P. et al., 'Obesity is associated with macrophage accumulation in adipose tissue', *Journal of Clinical Investigation*, 2003, vol. 112 (12): 1796-S08

16 Bjorbaek, C., Kahn, B.E., 'Leptin signaling in the central nervous system and the periphery', *Recent Progress in Hormone Research*, 2004, vol. 59: 305–31; Wang, Z.W. et al., 'The role of leptin resistance in the lipid abnormalities of aging', *FASEB Journal*, 2001, vol. 15 (l): 108–14; Bjorbaek, C. et al., 'The role of SOCS-3 in leptin signaling and leptin resistance', *Journal of Biological Chemistry*, 1999, vol. 274 (42): 30059–65; Wang, Z. et al., 'Leptin resistance of adipocytes in obesity: Role of suppressors of cytokine signaling', *Biochemistry and Biophysical Research Communications*, 14 October 2000, vol. 277 (1): 20–26; Bjorbaek, C. et al., 'Identification of SOCS-3 as a potential mediator of central leptin resistance', *Molecular Cell*, March 1998, vol. l (4): 619–25

17 Thomas, P., 'The big fat fix', *The Ecologist*, November 2006: 33–43

18 Sesso, H.D. et al., 'C-reactive protein and the risk of developing hypertension', *Journal of the American Medical Association*, 2003, vol. 290 (22): 2945–51

19 Blake, G.J., Ridker, P.M., 'Inflammatory biomarkers and cardiovascular risk prediction', *Journal of Internal Medicine*, 2002, vol. 252 (4): 283–94; Libby, P., Ridker, P.M., 'Inflammation and atherosclerosis: Role of c-reactive protein in risk assessment', *American Journal of Medicine*, 2004, vol. 116 (supplement 6A): 9S-16S

20 Seidel, S. et al., 'Assessment of commercial laboratories performing hair mineral analysis', *Journal of the American Medical Association*, 2001, vol. 285: 67–72

21 Colbin, A., *Food and Healing*, Ballantine, 1996

22 Mindell, E., *Shaping up with Vitamins*, Arlington, 1985

Chapter 7: The stress factor

1 McEwen, B.S., 'Protective and damaging effects of stress mediators', *New England Journal of Medicine*, 1998, vol. 338: 171–79

2 Seeman, T.E., Robbins, R.J., 'Aging and hypothalamic-pituitary-adrenal response to challenge in humans', *Endocrinology Review*, 1994, vol. 15: 233–60

3 Suzuki, T. et al., 'Low serum levels of dehydroepiandrosterone may cause deficient IL-2 production by lymphocytes in patients with systemic lupus erythematosus (SLE)', *Clinical and Experimental Innumology*, 1995, vol. 99: 251–55; Hedman, M. et al., 'Low blood and synovial fluid levels of sulpho-conjugated steroids in rheumatoid arthritis', *Clinical and Experimental Rheumatology*, 1992, vol. 10: 25–30

4 Brosschot, J.F. et al., 'Influence of life stress on immunological reactivity to mild psychological stress', *Psychosomatic Medicine*, 1994, vol. 56: 216–24

5 'Obesity and stress "hitting pets"', BBC News Online, 18 October 2004; online at: *http://news.bbc.co.uk/1/hi/uk/3751882.stm*

6 Everson, S.A. et al., 'Interaction of workplace demands and cardiovascular reactivity in progression of carotid atherosclerosis: Population based study', *British Medical Journal*, 1997, vol. 314: 553–38; Raikkonen, K. et al., 'Association of chronic stress with plasminogen activator inhibitor-1 in healthy middle-aged men', *Arteriosclerosis, Thrombosis and Vascular Biology*, 1996, vol. 16: 363–67

7 Vitaliano, P.P. et al., 'A path model of chronic stress, the metabolic syndrome, and coronary heart disease', *Psychosomatic Medicine*, 2002, vol. 64: 418–35

8 Stahl, F. et al., 'Dehydroepiandrosterone (DHEA) levels in patients with prostatic cancer, heart diseases and under surgery stress', *Experimental and Clinical Endocrinology*, 1992, vol. 99: 68–70; Donald, R.A. et al., 'Plasma corticotrophin releasing hormone, vasopressin, ACTH and cortisol responses to acute myocardial infarction', *Clinical Endocrinology*, 1994, vol. 40: 499–504

9 Lucini, D. et al., 'Hemodynamic and autonomic adjustments to real life stress conditions in humans', *Hypertension*, 2002, vol. 39: 184–88

10 Stoney, C.M., Engebretson, T.O., 'Plasma homocysteine concentrations are positively associated with hostility and anger', *Life Sciences*, 2000, vol. 66: 2267–75; Stoney, C.M., 'Plasma homocysteine levels increase in women during psychological stress', *Life Sciences*, 1999, vol. 64: 2359–65

11 Iso, H. et al., 'Perceived mental stress and mortality from cardiovascular disease among Japanese men and women: The Japan collaborative cohort study for evaluation of cancer risk sponsored by Monbusho (JACC Study)', *Circulation*, 2002, vol. 106: 1229–36

12 Laitinen, J. et al., 'Stress-related eating and drinking behavior and body mass index and predictors of this behavior', *Preventive Medicine*, 2002, vol. 34: 29–39; Vitaliano, V.T. et al., 'Insulin and glucose: Relationships with hassles, anger, and hostility in nondiabetic older adults', *Psychosomatic Medicine*, 1996, vol. 58: 489–99

13 Dallman, M.F. et al., 'Chronic stress and obesity: A new view of "comfort food"', *Proceedings of the National Academy of Sciences*, 2003, vol. 100 (20). 11696–701

14 Ibid.

15 Uno, H. et al., 'Hippocampal damage associated with prolonged and fatal stress in primates', *Journal of Neuroscience*,

1989, vol. 9: 1705–11; see also Sapolsky, R.M., *Stress, the Aging Brain and the Mechanisms of Neuron Death*, MIT Press, 1992

16 Cohen, J.H. et al., 'Psychological distress is associated with unhealthful dietary practices', *Journal of the America Dietetic Association*, 2002, vol. 102: 699–703

17 Galard, R. et al., 'Salivary cortisol levels and their correlation with plasma ACTH levels in depressed patients before and after the DST', *American Journal of Psychiatry*, 1991, vol. 148: 505-08; Anton, R.F., 'Urinary free cortisol in psychotic depression', *Biological Psychiatry*, 1987, vol. 22 (1): 24–34; von Zerssen, D. et al., 'Diurnal variation of mood and the cortisol rhythm in depression and normal states of mind', *European Archives of Psychiatry and Clinical Neuroscience*, 1987, vol. 237: 36–45

18 Guechot, J. et al., 'Physiological and pathological variations in saliva cortisol', *Hormone Research*, 1982, vol. 16: 357–64; Sachar, E.J. et al., 'Disrupted 24-hour patterns of cortisol secretion in psychotic depression', *Archives of General Psychiatry*, 1973, vol. 28: 19–24

19 Kaneko, M. et al., 'Hypothalamic-pituitary-adrenal axis function in chronic schizophrenia: Association with clinical features', *Neuropsychobiology*, 1992, vol. 25: 1–7

20 Lee, Y.H., Pratley, R.E., 'The evolving role of inflammation in obesity and the metabolic syndrome', *Current Diabetes Reports*, February 2005, vol. 5 (1): 70–75

21 Darmon, P. et al., 'Insulin resistance induced by hydrocortisone is increased in patients with abdominal obesity', *American Journal of Physiology-Endocrinology and Metabolism*, 2006, vol. 291: E995–E1002

22 Brindley, D.N., Rolland, Y., 'Possible connections between stress, diabetes, obesity, hypertension and altered lipoprotein metabolism that may result in atherosclerosis', *Clinical Science*, 1989, vol. 77: 453—61

23 Golding, J. et al., 'ALSPAC Study Team, ALSPAC – the Avon longitudinal study of parents and children. I. Study methodology', *Paediatric and Perinatal Epidemiology*, 2001, vol. 15: 74–87

24 Bosch, J.A. et al., 'Differential effects of active versus passive coping on secretory immunity', *Psychophysiology*, 2001, vol. 38: 836–46

25 Lee, S. et al., 'Prolonged exposure to intermittent alcohol vapors blunts hypothalamic responsiveness to immune and non-immune signals', *Alcoholism: Clinical and Experimental Research*, 2000, vol. 24: 110–22

26 Blumenthal, J.A. et al., 'Stress management and exercise training in cardiac patients with myocardial ischemia. Effects on prognosis and evaluation of mechanics', *Archives of Internal Medicine*, 1997, vol. 157: 2213–23

27 Surwit, R.S. et al., 'Stress management improves long-term glycemic control in type 2 diabetes', *Diabetes Care*, 2002, vol. 25: 30–34

28 Kirschbaum, C. et al., '"Normal" cigarette smoking increases free cortisol in habitual smokers', *Life Sciences*, 1992, vol. 50: 435–42; Kirschbaum, C., Hellhammer, D.H., 'Salivary cortisol in psychoneuroendocrine research: Recent developments and applications', *Psychoneuroendocrinology*, 1994, vol. 19: 313–33

29 Brissette, I. et al., 'The role of optimism in social network development, coping, and psychological adjustment during a life transition', *Journal of Personality and Social Psychology*, 2002, vol. 82: 102–11; Takkouche, B. et al., 'A cohort study of stress and the common cold', *Epidemiology*, 2001, vol. 11: 345–49

Chapter 8: You are what you eat

1 Gunderson, E.L., 'FDA total diet study, April 1982–April 1984: Dietary intakes of pesticides, selected elements, and other

chemicals', *Journal of the Association of Official Analytical Chemists* , 1988, vol. 71: 1200–09

2 Food and Drug Administration, *Total Diet Study: Summary of Residues found ordered by food, market baskets*, 91-3 to 99-1, FDA, September 2000

3 *Working Party on Pesticide Residues – 1999 Report*, MAFF Publications, 1999

4 *The 19th Australian Total Diet Survey*, Australia New Zealand Food Authority (ANZFA), April 2001

5 Environmental Working Group, *A Shopper's Guide to Pesticides in Produce*, EWG, 1995

6 Mayer, A.M., 'Historical changes in the mineral content of fruits and vegetables: A cause for concern?', *British Food Journal*, 1997, vol. 99: 207–11

7 McCance, R.A., Widdowson, E.M., *The Chemical Composition of Foods*, 1st edition, Special Report Series no: 235, Royal Society of Chemistry/MAFF, 1940; McCance, R.A., Widdowson, E.M., *The Chemical Composition of Foods*, 5th edition, Royal Society of Chemistry/MAFF, 1991

8 Thomas, D., 'Mineral depletion in foods over the period 1940 to 1991', *Nutrition Practice*, 2001, vol. 2: 27–29

9 'Vegetables without vitamins', no author listed, *Life Extension*, March 2001; online at: *www.lef.org/magazine/mag2001 /mar2001_report_vegetables.html*

10 Vines, G., 'Adipose is OK', *New Scientist*, 1995, vol. 146: 34–36; Pond, C.M., *The Fats of Life*, Cambridge University Press, 1998

11 Haas, E., *Staying Healthy With Nutrition*, Celestial Arts, 1992

12 Odelye, O. et al., 'Alcohol ingestion and lipoperoxidation: role of glutathione in antioxidant defense and detoxification', *Journal of Optimal Nutrition*, 1993, vol. 2: 173–89

13 Jones, D.P., 'Glutathione distribution in natural products: Absorption and tissue distribution', in Packer, L. (ed.), *Biothiols Methods in Enzymology*, vol. 252, Academic Press, 1995

14 Johnston, C.J. et al., 'Vitamin C elevates red blood cell glutathione in healthy adults', *American Journal of Clinical Nutrition*, 1993, vol. 58: 103–05

15 Snijder, M.B. et al., 'Adiposity in relation to vitamin D status and parathyroid hormone levels: A population-based study in older men and women', *Journal of Clinical Endocrinology & Metabolism*, 2005, vol. 90 (7): 4119–23; Ping-Delfos, W.C. et al., 'Acute suppression of food intake following dairy calcium and vitamin D', *Asia Pacific Journal of Clinical Nutrition*, 2004, vol. 13 (supplement): S82; Soares, M.J. et al., 'Dairy calcium and vitamin D stimulate postprandial thermogenesis: Effect in sequential meals', *Asia Pacific Journal of Clinical Nutrition*, 2004, vol. 13 (supplement): S56

16 Zhu, Y. et al., 'Calcium and 1 alpha, 25-dihydroxyvitamin D3 target TNF-alpha pathway to suppress experimental inflammatory bowel disease', *European Journal of Immunology*, 2005, vol. 35 (1): 217–24; Topilski, I. et al., 'The anti-inflammatory effects of 1,25-dihydroxyvitamin on TH2 cells in vivo are due in part to the control of integrin-mediated T lymphocyte homing', *European Journal of Immunology*, 2004, vol. 34 (4): 1068–76

17 Hayes, C.E. et al., 'The immunological functions of the vitamin D endocrine system', *Cellular and Molecular Biology*, 2003, vol. 49 (2): 277–300; Munger, K.L. et al., 'Vitamin D intake and incidence of multiple sclerosis', *Neurology*, 2004, vol. 62 (1): 60–65

18 Meydani, M. et al., 'Protective effect of vitamin E on exercise-induced oxidative damage in young and older adults', *American Journal of Physiology*, 1993, vol. 264: R992–98

19 Shakman, R.A., 'Nutritional influences on the toxicity of

environmental pollutants: A review', *Archives of Environmental Health*, 1974, vol. 28: 105–33

20 Zemal, M.B. et al., 'Calcium and dairy acceleration of weight and fat loss during energy restriction in obese adults', *Obesity Research*, 2004, vol. 12: 582–90

21 Clark, L.C. et al., 'Effects of selenium supplementation for cancer prevention in patients with carcinoma of the skin', *Journal of the American Medical Association*, 1996, vol. 276: 1957–63; Yoshizawa, K. et al., 'Study of prediagnostic selenium levels in toenails and the risk of advanced prostate cancer', *Journal of the National Cancer Institute*, 1998, vol. 90: 1219–24

22 Yoshida, M. et al., 'An evaluation of the bioavailability of selenium in high-selenium yeast', *Journal of Nutritional Science and Vitaminology*, 1999, vol. 45: 119–28

23 Erasmus, U., *Fats that Heal, Fats that Kill*, Alive Books, 1994

24 Holford, P., *The Optimum Nutrition Bible*, Piatkus, 1998

25 Pretty, J.N. et al., 'Farm costs and food miles: An assessment of the full cost of the UK weekly food basket', *Food Policy*, 2005, vol. 30: 1–19

26 Worthington, V., 'Nutritional quality of organic versus conventional fruits, vegetables and grains', *Journal of Alternative and Complementary Medicine*, 2001, vol. 7 (2): 161–73

Chapter 9: A menu for permanent weight loss

1 Won, D. et al., 'Indoor carpet as an adsorptive reservoir for volatile organic compounds', in *Proceedings of the 92nd Annual Meeting of the Air & Waste Management Association*, June 1999

2 Duehring, C., 'Carpet – EPA stalls and industry hedges while consumers remain at risk', *Informed Consent*, 1993, vol. 1: 6–32

3 Whitemore, R.W. et al., 'Non-occupational exposures to pesticides for residents of two U.S. cities', *Archives of*

Environmental Contamination and Toxicology, 1994, vol. 26: 47–59

4 Allsopp, M. et al., 'Hazardous Chemical In Carpets', Greenpeace Research Laboratories/University of Exeter, January 2001

5 Telles, S. et al., 'Physiological measures of right nostril breathing', *Journal of Alternative and Complementary Medicine*, 1996, vol. 2: 479–84; Telles, S. et al., 'Breathing through a particular nostril can alter metabolism and autonomic activities', *Indian Journal of Physiology & Pharmacology*, 1994, vol. 38: 133–37

6 Wood, C., 'Mood change and perceptions of vitality: A comparison of the effects of relaxation, visualization and yoga', *Journal of the Royal Society of Medicine*, 1993, vol. 86: 254–58

7 Telles, S., 'Oxygen consumption during pranayamic type of very slow-rate breathing', *Indian Journal of Medical Research*, 1991, vol. 94: 357–63

8 Bhatnagar, S.O., Jain, S.C., 'A study of response pattern on non-insulin-dependent diabetics to yoga therapy', *Diabetes Research & Clinical Practice*, 1993, vol. 19: 69–74

9 Boone, T., Flarity, J.R., 'Effects of qigong on cardiorespiratory changes: A preliminary study', *American Journal of Chinese Medicine*, 1993, vol. 21: 1–6

10 Pouls, M., 'Oral chelation and nutritional replacement therapy for chemical and heavy metal toxicity and cardiovascular disease', *Townsend Letter for Doctors and Patients*, 1999, vol. 192: 82–91

11 Foreman, H., 'Toxic side effects of EDTA', *Journal of Chronic Diseases*, 1963, vol. 16, 319–23

12 Halstead, B., 'The scientific basis of EDTA chelation therapy', *Life Enhancement*, February 1998, vol. 8

13 Pouls, M., 'Oral chelation and nutritional replacement

therapy for chemical and heavy metal toxicity and cardiovascular disease', *Townsend Letter for Doctors and Patients*, 1999, vol. 192: 82–91

14 Morita, K. et al., 'Chlorella accelerates dioxin excretion in rats', *Journal of Nutrition*, 1999, vol. 129: 1731–36

15 Tanaka, Y. et al., 'Studies on the inhibition of intestinal absorption of radioactive strontium, VI: Alginate degradation products as potent in vivo sequestering agents of radioactive strontium', *Canadian Medical Association Journal*, 1968, vol. 98: 1179–82

16 Connor, W.E., Connor, S.L., 'Should a low-fat, high-carbohydrate diet be recommended for everyone? The case for a low-fat, high-carbohydrate diet', *New England Journal of Medicine*, 1997, vol. 337: 562–68

17 Kekwick, A., Pawan, G.L.S., 'Calorie intake in relation to body-weight changes in the obese', *The Lancet*, 28 July 1956: 155–61

18 Tucker, L.A., Bagwell, M., 'Television viewing and obesity in adult females', *American Journal of Public Health*, 1991, vol. 81(7): 908–11; Tucker, L.A., Bagwell, M., 'Television viewing and obesity in adult males', *American Journal of Public Health*, 1989, vol. 79 (4): 516–18; Robinson, T.N., 'Reducing children's television viewing to prevent obesity', *Journal of the American Medical Association*, 1999, vol. 282: 1561–67

19 Crespo, C.J. et al., 'Television watching, energy intake, and obesity in US children: Results from the third national health and nutrition examination survey, 1988–1994', *Archives of Pediatric & Adolescent Medicine*, 2001, vol. 155: 360–65

20 Blair, S.N. et al., 'Changes in physical fitness and all-cause mortality. A prospective study of healthy and unhealthy men', *Journal of the American Medical Association*, 1995, vol. 273: 1093–98; Manson, J.E. et al., 'A prospective study of walking as

compared with vigorous exercise in the prevention of coronary heart disease in women', *New England Journal of Medicine*, 1999, vol. 341: 650–58

21 Steptoe, A. et al., 'The effects of exercise training on mood and perceived coping ability in anxious adults from the general population', *Journal of Psychosomatic Research*, 1989, vol. 33: 537–047; Blumenthal, J.A. et al., 'Effects of exercise training on older patients with major depression', *Archives of Internal Medicine*, 1999, vol. 159: 2349–56; Young, R.J., 'The effect of regular exercise on cognitive functioning and personality', *British Journal of Sports Medicine*, 1979, vol. 13: 110–17

22 Arroll, B., Beaglehole, R., 'Does physical activity lower blood pressure: A critical review of the clinical trials', *Journal of Clinical Epidemiology*, 1992; 45: 439–47

23 Hu, F.B. et al., 'Walking compared with vigorous physical activity and risk of type 2 diabetes in women: A prospective study', *Journal of the American Medical Association*, 1999, vol. 282: 1433–39

24 Ettinger, W.H., Jr, et al., 'A randomized trial comparing aerobic exercise and resistance exercise with a health education program in older adults with knee osteoarthritis', The Fitness Arthritis and Seniors Trial (FAST), *Journal of the American Medical Association*, 1997, vol. 277: 25–31

25 Martinez, M.E. et al., 'Leisure-time physical activity, body size, and colon cancer in women', Nurses' Health Study Research Group, *Journal of the National Cancer Institute*, 1997, vol. 89: 948–55; Giovannucci, E. et al., 'Physical activity, obesity, and risk for colon cancer and adenoma in men', *Annals of Internal Medicine*, 1995, vol. 122: 327–34

26 Aldoori, W.H. et al., 'Prospective study of physical activity and the risk of symptomatic diverticular disease in men', *Gut*, 1995, vol. 36: 276–82

27 Leitzmann, L.F. et al., 'Recreational physical activity and the risk of cholecystectomy in women', *New England Journal of Medicine*, 1999, vol. 341: 777–84

28 Campbell, A.J. et al., 'Randomised controlled trial of a general practice programme of home-based exercise to prevent falls in elderly women', *British Medical Journal*, 1997, vol. 315: 1065–69

29 King, A.C. et al., 'Moderate-intensity exercise and self-rated quality of sleep in older adults: A randomized controlled trial', *Journal of the American Medical Association*, 1997, vol. 277: 32–37; Montgomery, P., Dennis, J., 'Physical exercise for sleep problems in adults aged 60+ (Cochrane Review)', *Cochrane Database of Systematic Reviews*, 2002, vol. 4: CD003404

30 Biddle, S., 'Exercise and psychosocial health', *Research Quarterly for Exercise and Sport*, 1995, vol. 66: 292–97; Glenister, D., 'Exercise and mental health: A review', *Journal of the Royal Society for the Promotion of Health*, 1996, vol. 116: 7–13

31 Collingwood, T.R., Willett, L., 'The effects of physical training upon self-concept and body attitude', *Journal of Clinical Psychology*, 1971, vol. 27: 411–12

32 Skender, M.L. et al., 'Comparison of 2-year weight loss trends in behavioral treatments of obesity: Diet, exercise, and combination interventions', *Journal of the American Dietetic Association*, 1996, vol. 96: 342–46; Phinney, S.D., 'Exercise during and after very-low-calorie dieting', *American Journal of Clinical Nutrition*, 1992, vol. 56 (1 supplement): 190S–194S; Safer, D.J., 'Diet, behavior modification, and exercise: A review of obesity treatments from a long-term perspective', *Southern Medical Journal*, 1991, vol. 84: 1470–74

33 Pentimone, F., Del Corso, L., 'Why regular physical activity favors longevity', *Minerva Medica*, 1998, vol. 89: 197–201

34 Vistisen, K. et al., 'Cytochrome P450 IA2 activity in man measured by caffeine metabolism: Effect of smoking, broccoli and exercise', *Advances in Experimental Medicine and Biology*, 1991, vol. 283: 407–11; Moochhala, S.M. et al., 'Effects of acute physical exercise on aryl hydrocarbon hydroxylase activity in human peripheral lymphocytes', *Life Sciences*, 1990, vol. 47: 427–32

35 Kilburn, K.H. et al., 'Neurobehavioral dysfunction in firemen exposed to polycholorinated biphenyls (PCBs): Possible improvement after detoxification', *Archives of Environmental Health*, 1989, vol. 44: 345–50

36 Dunn, A.L. et al., 'Comparison of lifestyle and structured interventions to increase physical activity and cardiorespiratory fitness: A randomized trial', *Journal of the American Medical Association*, 1999, vol. 281: 327–34

37 Spelman, C.C. et al., 'Self-selected exercise intensity of habitual walkers', *Medicine & Science in Sports & Exercise*, 1993, vol. 25: 1174–79

38 Ginsburg, G.S. et al., 'Effects of a single bout of ultra-endurance exercise on lipid levels and susceptibility of lipids to peroxidation in triathletes', *Journal of the American Medical Association*, 1996, vol. 276: 221–25

39 Choi, B.M., Chung, H.T., 'Effect of qigong training on proportions of T lymphocyte subsets in human peripheral blood', *American Journal of Chinese Medicine*, 1995, vol. 23: 27–36; Choi, B.M., Chung, H.T., 'Delayed cutaneous hypersensitivity reactions in qigong trainees by multi-test, cell-mediated immunity', *American Journal of Chinese Medicine*, 1995, vol. 23: 139–44

40 MacIntosh, A., 'Exercise therapeutics update & commentary: Exercise and cortisol', *Townsend Letter for Doctors and Patients*, 1998, vol. 184: 38–40

41 Urhausen, A. et al., 'Impaired pituitary hormonal response to exhaustive exercise in overtrained endurance athletes', *Medicine & Science in Sports & Exercise*, 1998, vol. 30: 407–14

42 Paffenbarger, R.S. et al., 'The association of changes in physical-activity level and other lifestyle characteristics with mortality among men', *New England Journal of Medicine*, 25 February 1993, vol. 328 (8): 538–45; Sherman, S.E. et al., 'Physical activity and mortality in women in the Framingham Heart Study', *American Heart Journal*, November 1994, vol. 128 (5): 879–84; Lee, I.M. et al., 'Exercise intensity and longevity in men', *Journal of the American Medical Association*, 19 April 1995, vol. 273 (15): 1179–84; Lissner, L. et al., 'Physical activity levels and changes in relation to longevity: A prospective study of Swedish women', *American Journal of Epidemiology*, 1 January 1996, vol. 143 (1): 54–62

43 Young, R.J., 'The effect of regular exercise on cognitive functioning and personality', *British Journal of Sports Medicine*, 1979, vol. 13, 110–17

44 Morgan, W.P., 'Psychological effect of chronic physical activity', *Medicine & Science in Sports & Exercise*, 1970, vol. 2: 213–17

45 Griffin, S.J., Trinder, J., 'Physical fitness, exercise, and human sleep, *Psychophysiology*, 1978, vol. 15: 44–50

46 Collingwood, T.R., Willett, L., 'The effects of physical training upon self-concept and body attitude', *Journal of Clinical Psychology*, 1971, vol. 27: 411–12; Short, M.A. et al., 'Effects of physical conditioning on self-concept of adult obese males', *Physical Therapy*, February 1984, vol. 64 (2): 194–98

47 Goñi, A., Zulaika, L., 'Relationships between physical education classes and the enhancement of fifth grade pupils' self-concept', *Perceptual & Motor Skills*, August 2000, vol. 91 (1): 246–50

48 Goto, K. et al., 'Enhancement of fat metabolism by repeated bouts of moderate endurance exercise', *Journal of Applied Physiology*, June 2007, vol. 102 (6): 2158–64

49 Kleiner, S.M., 'Water: An essential but overlooked nutrient', *Journal of the American Dietetic Association*, 1999, vol. 99: 200–06

50 Valtin, H., 'Drink at least eight glasses of water a day. Really? Is there scientific evidence for "8 x 8"?', *American Journal of Physiology. Regulatory, integrative and comparative physiology*, 2002, vol. 283: R993–R1004

51 Tobin, R.S. et al., 'Effects of activated carbon and bacteriostatic filters on microbiological quality of drinking water', *Applied and Environmental Microbiology*, 1981, vol. 41: 646–51

52 Daschner, F.D. et al., 'Microbiological contamination of drinking water in a commercial household water filter system', *European Journal of Clinical Microbiology & Infectious Diseases*,1996, vol. 15: 233–37

53 'Bottling out', no author credited, *The Ecologist*, February 2003, vol. 46

54 Hurst, D.F. et al., 'The relationship of self-esteem to the health-related behaviors of the patients of a primary care clinic', *Archives of Family Medicine*, 1997, vol. 6: 67–70

55 Pascucci, M.A., Loving, G.L., 'Ingredients of an old and healthy life: A centenarian perspective', *Journal of Holistic Nursing*, 1997, vol. 15: 199–213

56 Swan, G.E., Carmelli, D., 'Curiosity and mortality in aging adults: A 5-year follow-up of the Western Collaborative Group Study', *Psychology and Aging*, 1996, vol. 11: 449–53

57 Friedman, H.S. et al., 'Does childhood personality predict longevity?', *Journal of Personality and Social Psychology*, 1993, vol. 65: 176–85

58 Lawton, M.P. et al., 'A two-factor model of caregiving appraisal and psychological well-being', *Journal of Gerontology*, 1991, vol. 46: 181–89

59 Woodward, W., 'New surprises in very old places: Civil War nurse leaders and longevity', *Nursing Forum*, 1991, vol. 26: 9–16

Index

adaptive thermogenesis 81, 82

adaptogens 153–4

addiction 126–9, 135

additives 41, 121, 122, 124–5, 166–7, 182

adipocytes *see* fat cells

adipokines 130

adrenaline (epinephrine) 32, 82, 146, 204

aerobic exercise 202–3

age, and incidence of obesity 54

air conditioning 54

air fresheners 95, 122

alcohol 46, 67, 69, 70, 136–7, 154

allergies 55, 121–39

    and addiction 126–9, 135

    and inflammation 129–32

    and sleep problems 66–7, 71

    tests 132–4, 199

    toxins and 83, 90

    and weight gain 125–6, 128

animal fats 95

animals

    antibiotic treatment 106, 111–12, 115

    meat production 165–7

    stress 144–5

anorexia 28

antibiotics 106, 111–12, 113, 115, 117, 167

antibodies 132–4, 199

antidepressants 54, 69, 103, 104, 106–8, 114

antihypertensives 108–9

antioxidants 175, 182, 193, 194

antipsychotics 108

appetite control 34, 64, 82

autoimmune diseases 34, 47, 90, 130, 188

'bad' food 159–61

basal metabolic rate (BMR) 20–1, 43, 81–2

beans 194

benzodiazepines 69

benzopyrene 85–6

beta-blockers 104–5, 109

binge-eating 29, 148, 197

bisphenol-A 83, 85, 92–3

blood, toxins in 76–7

blood groups 128–9

blood-sugar levels 32, 34, 63, 70–1, 78, 125

body fat *see* fat cells

Body Mass Index (BMI) 12, 24, 26–7, 59, 61

bone problems 10, 17, 29, 202

brain

    role in weight control 33, 63

    sleep debt and 59

breakfast 161, 162

breast cancer 10, 47–8, 58, 72, 89

breathing 190–1

bulimia 28

C-reactive protein (CRP) 132

cadmium 86, 93, 94, 191

caffeine 66, 69, 70, 72, 163

calcium 29, 71, 138, 154, 173, 177, 182

calories 18–21, 42–4

cancer 10, 187, 188

    breast 10, 47–8, 58, 72, 89

    colon 35

    diet and 121

    drugs 117

    light levels and 72

    toxins and 88, 90, 95

car exhausts 93

carbamates 84

carbohydrates 70–1, 121, 136, 147, 162–3, 196–7

carbonated drinks 40

carpets 188–9

cells *see* fat cells

chelation therapy 191–3

chemicals *see* toxins

chemotherapy drugs 117

children

    dieting 20–1

    drugs 107, 108

    environmental toxins 89–90, 189

    heredity 55

    junk food 182

    obesity 25–6, 45

    sleep debt 59–60, 61–2

    stress/weight gain cycle 149

    television viewing 198

    toxins and 89–90

China 40

chocolate 139, 163, 165

chromium 182

chronic illness 29

cigarettes *see* smoking

class differences 44–6

climate 51–2

coffee 136–7, 163

colon cancer 35

'comfort food' 146–7

constipation 29

contraceptive drugs 54, 92, 104, 110, 111, 116–17

convenience foods 161, 163

cooking 182–3

copper 173

cortisol 32, 63, 143–4, 145, 146, 147–9, 154–5, 202

cosmetics 94

cravings 108, 110, 126, 127, 134–9, 160, 184, 197

dairy products 136–7, 163

darkness, and insomnia 72–3

DDT and DDE 77, 80, 81, 88, 164–5

depression 10, 69, 102, 105, 106–8, 139, 147–8

detoxification 97–100, 200

developing countries 39–40, 44

DHEA 143

diabetes 10, 16

    drug-induced 109

    drug treatment 54, 102, 104, 109–10

    gestational diabetes 55

    sleep debt and 53, 59, 62–3, 64

    toxins and 78

dieting 11

    calories in/calories out 18–21, 22

children 20–1
diet industry 22–6, 28
effects of dieting culture 27–9
eliminating food groups 21–2
failure of 11, 15–16, 23
menu for permanent weight loss 185–209
rebound effect 11, 19–21, 82
releasing toxins 76–7
sleep and weight loss 65–6
digestion 62, 205
dioxins 94, 167
diuretics 97, 109
DNA 51
drinks
caffeinated 66
carbonated 40
sports drinks 206–7
water 204–8
driving, reaction times 29–30
drugs 54, 101–18
in animal feed 167
in the environment 111–12
for insomnia 69
sleep disruption 105–6
in water supply 112–18

eating disorders 28–9, 127
eating habits 40, 146, 180–4
economics, diet industry 23
EDTA 192–3
eicosapentaenoic acid (EPA) 178
endocrine system *see* hormones

energy, sleep debt and 66

enkephalin 127

environmental toxins 39, 90–6, 111–12, 151–2,
    186–9

epinephrine (adrenaline) 32, 82, 146, 204

essential fatty acids (EFAs) 178–80

ethnic groups 46, 54

European Union 23

exercise 11, 41–4, 99, 153, 200–4

fast food 40–1, 183

fasting 98–100

fat cells

    distribution of 31–2

    functions 30

    hormone receptors 82

    and inflammation 131

    leptin and 32–6

    stress hormones and 148

    toxins stored in 53–4, 76, 81, 83

fats

    animal fats 95

    healthy fats 178–80

fertility 10, 55, 187

fertilizers 172–3

fibre 29, 194

flame-retardants 85, 96, 189

flea collars 95

fluid retention 76, 110, 125, 128

food

    additives 41, 121, 122, 124–5, 166–7, 182

    allergies 71, 121–39

'bad' food 159–61
and cancer 121
carbohydrates 196–7
'comfort food' 146–7
cravings 108, 110, 126, 127, 134–9, 160, 184, 197
and detoxification 97
diet foods 23, 28
eating habits 40, 146, 180–4
fads 160–1
food intolerance 71, 76, 122, 134
'functional foods' 193–5
healthy eating 162–3
healthy fats 178–80
juices 195–6
junk food 40–1, 182
local food 180–1
missing nutrients 172–4
organic food 168–9, 181–2
pesticide residues 95–6, 163–72
shopping for 46
tinned food 92–3
toxins in 163–72
water content 206
formaldehyde 186
fractures, hip 17–18
free radicals 68, 145, 175, 182
fruit 121
fasting 99
'functional foods' 194
healthy eating 162, 163
juices 195

   missing nutrients 172–4

   organic food 182

   pesticide residues 164–5, 168–72

'functional foods' 193–5

garlic 194

gastric bypasses 81

genetics 38–9, 47–52

geographical location, and obesity 12–13, 87–8

ghrelin 63–4

globalization 40

glutathione 175–6

grains 96, 197

'grazing' 41

green foods 97, 162

healthy eating 162–3

heart, fat deposits around 31–2

heart disease 10, 34, 68, 90, 102, 145–6, 154

herbicides 174

herbs 71–2, 98, 153–4, 195, 196

high blood pressure 10, 68

   drugs 54, 104–5, 107, 108–9

   sleep debt and 59

   stress and 145

hip fractures 17–18

histamine 123, 132

Hong Kong 40

hormones

   body fat and 30, 32

   functions 78

   hormone replacement therapy (HRT) 92

and inflammation 130–1

leptin 32–6

pollution and 53–4, 78–82

relaxation and 68

sleep debt and 53, 58, 59, 62–4

steroids 110–11

stress hormones 32, 63, 68, 141–9

toxins and 78–82

in water supply 113, 116–17

hunger 125–6

hypertension *see* high blood pressure

hypothalamus 33, 63

IMED 127

immune system

allergies 122–3, 127

effects of stress 142–3, 150

leptin and 34

sleep and 58

toxins and 90

India 40

industrial chemicals *see* toxins

infant formula 93

infertility 10, 187

inflammation 55, 83, 129–32

insomnia 68–70

insulin

carbohydrates and 196–7

and inflammation 130, 131

sleep and 53, 62–3

stress and 149

and weight gain 102, 104, 109–10

Inuit 52
iron 29, 139, 154, 173–4, 182

juices 195–6
junk food 40–1, 182

kidneys 97, 100, 205

lead 86, 191, 192
lectins 128
leptin 32–6, 49, 63–4, 67, 129, 130–1, 149
lifestyle, urban 39–40
light, artificial 58, 72–3
linoleic acid 178
lipids 31
liver 97, 100
local food 180–1
low-calorie diets 15

macrophages 131
magnesium 21, 71, 138, 139, 154, 173, 177, 182
mattresses 71
meat 106, 112, 161, 163, 165–7, 173, 183, 186
melatonin 58, 62, 72–3
memory, stress and 147
menopause 17
menstrual problems 10, 29, 188
menstruation 149
mercury 87, 91, 192, 193
Metabolic Syndrome 59, 64, 65, 148
metabolism
    dieting and 20–1

    drugs and 104

    exercise and 43

    sleep and 62–4

    toxins and 76, 78–9, 80–3

metals

    chelation therapy 191–3

    'functional foods' 194, 195

    testing for 198–9

microwave ovens 182–3

minerals

    chelation therapy 193

    missing nutrients 172–4

    organic food 182

    stress reduction 154

    supplements 174–5, 177–8

    testing for 199

mitochondrial DNA 51

moods, stress and 147

mortality rates 17–18, 25

mothers, age of 54

muscles

    exercise 201, 203

    fat deposits 32

    loss of 43

    low-calorie diets 21

nappies, disposable 94–5

nervous system 30, 65, 82, 142–3

noradrenaline (norepinephrine) 82, 146

nutritional medicine 121–2

nutritional supplements 174–8

obesity and overweight

    allergies and 125–6, 128

    in children 25–6, 45

    definition of 24

    drugs and 102–11

    exercise and 41–4

    genetic factors 47–52

    and geographical location 12–13, 87–8

    health consequences 10

    increase in prevalence 9–10

    inflammation and 130–1

    junk food and 40–1

    mortality rates 17–18, 25

    in pets 144–5

    sleep debt and 59–61

    social class and 44–6

    as stand-alone disease 25

    stress and 148–9

    toxins and 78–88

    urban lifestyle and 39–40

oestrogen 110, 149

    after menopause 17

    as animal growth-promoter 112

    contraceptive pill 92

    hormone replacement therapy (HRT) 92

    soya-based infant formula 93

    toiletries and 94

    in water supply 116–17

omega-3 fatty acids 178–9

omega-6 fatty acids 178–80

onions 194

organic food 168–9, 181–2

organochlorines 81–3, 88

organophosphates 84, 95

organotins 83, 84–5

osteoporosis 17, 29, 34, 202

overweight *see* obesity and overweight

oxidative stress 201–2

oxygen 190–1, 201–2

paper products 94

parabens 94

PCBs 77, 81, 88, 98, 167, 195, 200

pectin 194

perfumes 95, 122

pesticides 81–2, 84, 91, 95–6, 113, 115, 164–5, 167–72, 189

pharmaceutical industry 23–4

phenobarbital 89

phosphorus 138, 174

phthalates 85, 92–5

pollution 13, 75–100

    children and 89–90, 189

    detoxification 97–100, 200

    drugs in the environment 111–12

    environmental toxins 39, 90–6, 111–12, 151–2, 186–9

    geographical location and 87–8

    hormones 53–4, 78–82

    in food 95–6, 163–72

    reducing exposure to 90–6

    weight gain and 80–6

polybrominated flame-retardants 85

portion sizes 162

potassium 138, 154, 174

poverty 44, 45

pregnancy 55, 114

processed foods 41

progesterone 110–11, 149

prostaglandins 178

prostate cancer 95

protein 21, 163, 183

puberty 35, 149

reaction times 29–30

rebound weight gain 11, 19–21, 82

relaxation 67–8, 70

rest 203

Ritalin 89

salt 121, 136–7, 163, 184

saunas 98

seasonal food 183

seaweeds 195

selenium 154, 175, 177–8

serotonin 71, 146–7

set point, metabolism 20–1, 78

sewage 115–16

shopping, social class and 46

showers 114–15

skipped meals 20

sleep 53, 57–73

    drug disruption 105–6

    how to get to sleep 70–3

    insomnia 68–70

    metabolic regulation 62–4

and obesity 59–61

snoring 64–5, 66–7

television and 61–2

and weight loss 65–6

smoking 46, 54, 70, 71, 89, 94, 126–7, 154–5

snacks 40–1, 70–1

snoring 64–5, 66–7

social class 44–6

SOCS 131

sodium 174

solvents 86, 113

soya products 93

sports 43–4

sports drinks 206–7

starvation 10, 35

steroids 54, 103, 104, 105, 110–11, 112, 114

stress 71, 141–55

in animals 144–5

beneficial stress 150–1

environmental stress 151–2

and mental problems 147–8

stress hormones 32, 63, 68, 141–9

stress management 152–5

and weight gain 146–7

strokes 16, 145–6

sugar 135, 136–7, 163, 184

sulphur 154, 194

sunscreens 94

supplements 174–8

sweating 98

Syndrome X *see* Metabolic Syndrome

tampons 94

tea 163, 195

television 55, 61–2, 96, 198

temperatures 54

thiazolidinediones (TZDs) 109, 110

thighs, fat deposits 32

thyroid hormones 63, 79, 81

thyroid problems 78, 96

tinned food 92–3

toiletries 94, 99

toxins 75–100

    in animal feed 167

    children and 89–90

    detoxification 97–100, 200

    drugs as 105

    effect on metabolism 80–3

    environmental toxins 39, 90–6, 111–12, 151–2,

        186–9

    in food 163–8

    and hormones 78–82

    testing for 198–9

    types of 84–6

tranquillizers 69, 72, 113

underweight, health risks 17

United States of America, industrial areas 87–8

urban lifestyle 39–40

urine 205

vegetables 121, 162

    fasting 99

    'functional foods' 194–5

juices 195–6
missing nutrients 172–4
organic food 182
pesticide residues 96, 164–5, 168–72
vitamins
  chelation therapy 193
  cravings for 138
  missing nutrients 172–4
  organic food 182
  stress reduction 154
  supplements 174–5, 176–7
  vitamin B complex 21, 71, 138, 154,
    176
VOCs (volatile organic compounds) 91, 97, 187,
  188–9

walking 201, 203
water 204–8
  antibiotic residues 106
  bottled water 207–8
  drugs in 112–18
  filters 118, 207
  toxins in 92, 186–7
  while fasting 99
weight gain
  allergies and 125–6, 128
  drugs and 102–11
  in middle age 17–18
  problems of fluctuating 16
  rebound effect 11, 19–21, 82
  and stress 146–7
  see also obesity

weight loss *see* dieting
willpower 38

yo-yo dieting 16, 20–1, 76–7

zinc 154, 173, 175, 177